Breasts

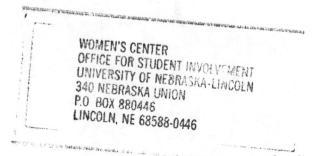

Breasts
Our Most Public Private Parts

MEEMA SPADOLA

WILDCAT CANYON PRESS
A Division of Circulus Publishing Group, Inc.
Berkeley, California

Breasts: Our Most Public Private Parts
Copyright © 1998 by Meema Spadola
Cover photographs copyright © 1998 by Isa Brito

Publisher: Julienne Bennett
Editor: Roy M. Carlisle
Copyeditors: Carol Rhodes and Holly A. Taines
Cover Design: Big Fish Design
Interior Design: Gordon Chun Design
Typesetting: Holly A. Taines
Typographic Specifications: Body text set in 11/18 Berkeley Book. Cos-
mos Medium is used for display.

Printed in the United States of America
Cataloging-in-Publication Data
Spadola, Meema, 1969–
     Breasts : our most public private parts / Meema Spadola.
          p. cm.
     Includes bibliographical references (pp. 245-247).
     ISBN 1-885171-27-7 (pbk. : alk. paper)
     1. Breasts—Social aspects. 2. Breasts—Psychological aspects.
3. Body image in women. I. Title.
GT498.B74S63   1998
391.6—dc21   98-39138   CIP

Distributed to the trade by Publishers Group West
10 9 8 7 6 5 4 3 2 1

To my family,
whose love and support mean the world to me—
especially Mom and Granny.

Author's Notes

1. Hearing women's stories is powerful, but seeing real women's everyday breasts is also an important part of coming to terms with our own bodies. For this reason, the publisher and I encourage women to supplement the reading of this book by watching the video, *Breasts: A Documentary*.

2. Some individuals' names have been changed and certain characteristics disguised in order to protect contributors' privacy.

3. While the ideas and suggestions about breast health contained in this book are intended to inform, they should not be substituted for consulting with a physician. I strongly encourage women to discuss breast health issues with their physicians and other medical professionals.

4. The names of many products mentioned in these pages are registered trademarks, belonging to their owners. I include mention of them as they enhance various stories, and I acknowledge the rights of their owners.

Acknowledgments

Neither books nor films are made by one person alone. Without the documentary *Breasts*, I never would have written this book. Thom Powers, my creative partner and friend—it's been a great adventure so far. I can't thank you enough for pushing me to start this project and for being there to help me all the way. Thanks to Rocky Collins at Elevator Pictures who gave his time, advice, and equipment to help make *Breasts* possible. To our amazing crew: Ann Moore, our editor, who truly helped shaped *Breasts*; Eileen Schreiber, our director of photography; and John Davis, Ananda Ellis, and Rehana Ellis for the music. To others at Elevator Pictures: Steve Apicella, Annetta Marion, Moon Cho, Carol Stutz, and Jim Lovaglio who provided continual support. To Cynthia Hsiung, who presented the project to HBO; and to the great team at HBO/Cinemax: Sheila Nevins, Jackie Glover, and Jonathan Moss, who brought *Breasts* to television viewers. Thanks also to Henry McGee and Cynthia Rhea at HBO Home Video, and Jan Rofekamp at Films Transit.

I'm lucky to be surrounded by friends, family, and colleagues who inspire and support me—particularly through the documentary and in writing this book. Thanks especially to

Dad and Nancy, Mom and Amy, and my brother, Emilio who have helped in so many ways. I am grateful for friends like Risa Mickenberg, for her constant enthusiasm and her reading and discussion of chapters, and to Steve Kessler, as well, for letting us shoot *Breasts* photos at their home; Leela Jacinto, for her insightful editorial assistance; Julie Besonen, for her help in shaping the original proposal. Keira Alexandra, Jonathan Diamond, Joe Dorman, Amy Einhorn, Rolfe Kent, Chris Lindsay Abaire, Rebecca Lorins, Leslie Mello, Stephen Metcalf, Daniel Polin, Debbie Stoller, Olivier Sultan, Paul Tough, John Walter, Sasha Waters, Koethi Zan, and Carolina Zorrilla de San Martin all helped support me and *Breasts* in one way or another. Thanks also to Jodi Sh. Doff, my speedy transcriber; and my research assistants: Haley Collazo, Westry Green, Tannie Huang, and Pamela Lund. And much gratitude to Shelley Studenberg, who kept my wrists, back, and neck functioning.

I extend thanks also to my editor, Roy M. Carlisle and the entire Circulus Publishing Group, Inc./Wildcat Canyon Press staff, especially Holly, Aimee, Leyza, and Rose who encouraged their bosses to publish this book. Much gratitude to Holly A. Taines and Carol Rhodes for their copyediting. Thanks to my agent, Sharon Friedman, who loved this idea from the start. And to photographer Isa Brito, who was a joy to work with and helped make this project truly collaborative.

Most of all, I thank the women and girls who shared their stories and their breasts with me. You inspire and move me.

• • • • •

The Story of Our Breasts

I believe that every woman has a breast story—and I don't mean a story *about* her breasts. I mean the story *of* her breasts. The premise is simple: Breasts are the most public private part of our bodies. As women we are simultaneously told that we must hide our breasts (in some states, simply breast feeding in public is an arrestable offence), and show them off (after all, breasts are part of what make us sexy as women). But, of course, whether we cover them or flaunt them, our breasts are right there—their approximate size is public knowledge. No one can deny that our breasts play a crucial role in our experiences of puberty, motherhood, sex, health, and aging. So it's logical that how we feel about our breasts can profoundly impact our lives. Yet when is the last time you heard women—ordinary women of all ages, sizes, and backgrounds—speak honestly and openly about what their breasts mean to them?

Since the beginning of history, breasts have been measured, examined, put on display, and commented on by men. But what if women started to talk and ask each other about how our breasts have shaped our lives? Hearing a woman share her terror of finding a lump in her breast, or a mother talk about the pains and pleasures of breast feeding, or a seventy-five-year-old woman speak about watching her breasts grow older, can open the door to a wide range of discussion. And through this, we just might learn something about what it means to be a woman, or a pubescent girl; what it means to have breast cancer, or breast feed, or grow older. We might better understand how we think about our sexuality and how we see our bodies in relation to ourselves and to our partners.

Think for a minute about what we *do* hear about breasts. Much has been said about the barrage of breasts in commercials, magazines, television shows, and movies. While we all complain about the role of the media, I think it's important to remember that we buy what the media machine is selling. We might want to ask ourselves why it is that we only see one kind of breasts: perfectly round, firm, perky, and young—not too big, not too small. Yet how many of us fit into that category? Countless magazine articles tell us what we should look like and how we should feel about our breasts, but few of us find these comforting or even very informative. And many of us seem to have little faith in our doctors either. Many women report that their doctors are rarely willing or able to answer their questions, and often, we are uncomfortable asking.

Where is the unbiased and accurate information about breasts? Beyond medical or fashion advice, we need stories against which we can realistically measure ourselves—literally and figuratively. Because most of us rarely see other women's bodies, we have a fairly warped view of what constitutes "normal" breasts. It makes perfect sense. If we see only our un-airbrushed breasts in comparison to a steady diet of movie and magazine breasts (which benefit from makeup, lighting, photo touch-ups, impossibly long hours at the gym, and often, surgery), our own real breasts don't fare so well. We simply don't see stretch marks, nipple hair, mastectomies, or lopsided, saggy breasts. Dr. Loren Eskenazi, a plastic surgeon in San Francisco, told me that she became concerned when her clients told her that they just wanted "normal" breasts. She'd look at normal pair after normal pair, and know that what they were asking for were, in fact, the fairly unusual breasts that we're told are the ideal. Hoping to share with her clients her own knowledge of the normal variations that occur, she began compiling a catalog of photographs of women's naked torsos to chart the breasts of hundreds of women of all ages, shapes, and sizes. If only this kind of realistic view of our breasts were available to every woman who believes that she isn't "normal."

My own breast story certainly doesn't begin with this book. It's hard for me to pinpoint the exact time in my life that I started thinking about breasts, but I do know that early on I picked up on the fact that they were the most outward sign of being a woman. More than anything, I looked forward to growing up and having breasts. Even the simple ritual of putting on a bra seemed to contain some wonderful and secret knowledge. (Would I ever learn to hook a bra behind my back?) When I was nine, my best friend and I went to ballet class together where we wore little pink tights and black leotards. I was so envious of her newly developing breasts. Once, I cried to her, "Why am I so flat and you're so fluffy?" She put her arm around me and comforted me saying, "It's not as great as you think it is." And she was right. She developed far too quickly, and though we were the same height in our teen years, she was a D-cup and I was an A. She had her growth spurt early— I had to wait until college for mine. Ironically, we ended up about the same size when she got a breast reduction at the end of high school. Looking back, I know that even though I ended up with a perfectly normal-sized pair of breasts, for years the sense of not having enough, and perhaps not being enough of a woman, stuck with me. All through high school and college, breast size was a popular discussion topic, and I was always amazed at how much my friends' breasts had affected their perceptions of themselves as women. What other body part is that powerful?

In 1995, I decided to make a documentary film that would explore how women's breasts shape their lives. Working with my co-producer, Thom Powers, I circulated questionnaires around New York City asking women to tell us about their breasts. The response was overwhelming. After sorting through over two hundred questionnaires, letters, phone messages, and photographs, I chose my interviewees. During one particularly hot, humid weekend in July 1995, we gathered the women in a small studio in Manhattan. One by one or in pairs, women sat down on a stool in front of our all-female crew and told me their breast stories. The atmosphere during the shoot was unlike any other I've experienced. Interviewees arrived at the studio understandably anxious—after all, I had asked them to appear topless during their interviews. But as the day progressed, the film crew and the interviewees grew more comfortable, and debated, laughed, and shared serious stories about their breasts during breaks in the shooting.

When we completed the film, twenty-two women and

girls were represented—ranging in age from six to eighty-four years old. Many of them were topless (with the exception of the younger interviewees, of course), but all of them bared more than just their breasts. Their candid thoughts were humorous, moving, and often surprising. Among the original interviewees are two sisters, ages six and ten; an eleven year old on the verge of puberty; a mother with her infant daughter at her breast; two strippers with implants; two women with mastectomies; a woman with silicone implants that she fears have damaged her health; the self-proclaimed leader of "The Strong Breast Revolution;" a beautiful transsexual; a 420-pound comedienne with "wraparound" breasts; and two mother/daughter pairs.

What began as an independent project received finishing funds from the HBO-owned channel Cinemax, which has a series, "Reel Life," committed to showing new documentaries. When *Breasts* premiered in January 1997, it was the highest rated documentary ever aired on "Reel Life." And despite some initial concern about how critics might react to such an unusual film, the reviews were positive. Clearly people were intrigued by the premise, and once they tuned in, they had a chance to hear stories they never expected.

When I began the film, I had no idea that so many women would be so eager to discuss their feelings about their breasts. I worried that my theory was based only on my and a few of my closest friends' unique experiences. But since then, I've realized that as women we'd never been given an opportunity to talk about our breasts, and now that we've started talking, we don't want to stop. During the three years since I began this project, I have spoken to hundreds of women who tell me essentially the same thing: Whether our story begins in childhood (perhaps as a fascination with our mother nursing a younger sibling), in puberty during development, because of a sexual experience (positive or negative), in pregnancy and motherhood, or because of a health problem, at some point, our breasts will shape how we look at the world, and how the world looks back at us.

In writing *Breasts*, I spoke to nearly two hundred additional women and girls from all over the country. The youngest was two, the oldest ninety—in between there are women and girls of all ages, shapes, sizes, and backgrounds. (I often identify women with both age and cup size, and for brevity's sake I describe women as *being* a 34B, for example, rather than "having 34B breasts.")

My qualifications for writing a book on breasts comes from having two of them, thinking about breasts for years, and hearing the breast stories of hundreds of women. But this book is by no means intended to be the end of the discussion on breasts. Rather, I'd love to see readers use it as a catalyst for telling their own breast stories, and for encouraging the women in their lives to share theirs. Perhaps some of you will be inspired to share your accounts with us. Certainly, while there are common themes in the stories I've heard, each woman's experience is unique. I'd love for breasts to stop being seen *only* as sexual, or for nursing a child, or feared because of the threat of cancer. How freeing it would be if we could see breasts in all of their complexity. Many women have told me that after watching the documentary—hearing the women's stories and seeing their very real breasts—they felt better about their own bodies. I hope that this book will do the same for readers. Some of these women's experiences will seem familiar to you, others may be difficult to imagine, but I do hope that they'll spark some of your own memories and feelings. I know that working on this project has positively affected how I look at my breasts, and by extension, my entire body and sense of myself as a woman.

apples, babaloos, bags, bazongas, bazooms, Berthas, bies, boob bits, breas buffers, bumpers, bust, cans, cantaloupes, cassabas, cat and kitties, catheads, cha chas, charlies, charms, chest, chestnuts, cliff, coconuts, cups, dairies, diddies, dinners, doorknobs, droopers, dumplings, eyes, fried eggs, gazombas, globes, gondolas, grapefruits, ha has, Harry and Junes, headlights, hooters, ice cream scoops, jerseycities, jugs, kajoobies, knobs, knockers, lemons, love pillows, lungs, mammae, mammary glands, maracas, marshmallow mountains, melons, milk bottles, milkers, mosquito bites, nice ones, nipples, nips, orbs, pair, pancakes, peaches, pumps, puppies with the pink noses, rack, second pair of eyes, snack trays, sweater meat, ta tas, teats, the girls, tits, titties, tomatoes, torpedoes, twins, udders, upper frontal superstructure, walnuts, water balloons, watermelons, whales

CHILDHOOD

You'll need a calculator for this joke: *Dolly Parton went to the doctor and he measured her breasts. They were sixty-nine inches around* (punch in 69) *and he said, "Dolly! That is too, too, too much!"* (punch in 222). *So he gave her fifty-one pills* (punch in 51) *to take eight times a day* (hit the multiplication sign and 8). *And* (now press the equal sign and turn the calculator upside down), *she woke up "BOOBLESS!"*

—Popular elementary school joke, circa 1980

When twenty-five-year-old Dallas was a little girl in Maine, she and her friends used to take her mother's bras and stuff socks in them to do can-can routines. They called themselves "The Boob Shakers." Carol, twenty-one, grew up in a tight-knit extended family in which "someone was always breast feeding." Her fantasy games consisted of breast feeding her dolls and she dreamed of having big breasts. Growing up in Indiana, Jane, forty-four, wanted to look like the photograph of Marilyn Monroe in her father's *Playboy*. Zoe, twenty-five, remembers watching her mother use her breasts as a sexual tool. "She would flirt with her boyfriends, brushing her breasts against them." And when I was little, I tried on my mother's bras, stuffing them to achieve the desired effect. I couldn't imagine

3

how a woman could reach behind her back and fasten her bra each and every day. I'd watch my mother slip on her bra, hooking it in the back. (She didn't fasten it in front, then turn it around, as I did.) Then she'd bend over and scoop her breasts up in the bra. I'd do the same, though I had nothing to scoop. I wanted more than anything to have something to fill my very own bra.

As children we're like detectives busily learning about our bodies and the world around us, picking up clues from our family, friends, and the media about what breasts mean. We discover right away that breasts are powerful—whether they're associated with sex or mothering—and we learn that all breasts are not created equal. Even as very small children, our attitudes about breasts fit neatly into the classic mother versus whore paradigm: breasts are either comforting or sexual. Even if we don't remember these early influences, what we learn about breasts during this period affects our whole lives.

Childhood games and toys help shape our attitudes. In her book *Forever Barbie*, M.G. Lord explores the history of Barbie and the impact she has had on millions of little girls since her appearance in 1959. "Barbie was a revelation. . . . She was all that we could be and—if you calculate what at human scale would translate to a thirty-nine-inch bust—more than we could be," writes Lord.[1] Carol, who was born in Puerto Rico and grew up in the Bronx, was surrounded by blonde Barbies as a little girl. "Every Christmas, birthday, or Easter, I could count on getting a Barbie. It was the staple gift for the girls in my family. The runner-up was a Cabbage Patch Kid. We had Barbie to see what we should look like, and a Cabbage Patch Kid to practice what we should be: a mother. Growing up with Barbie negatively influenced my body-image, yet where else could I see a woman who could be anything she wanted (Doctor Barbie, Pilot Barbie, Businesswoman Barbie)?"

I was one of the few girls to grow up Barbie-free. I did have a doll, but she was just a baby doll, entirely unlike womanly Barbie—tall, slim, blonde, with long legs and high, hard, nippleless breasts. And then there was Skipper—Barbie's far less glamorous, brunette, and flat-chested sidekick. In 1975 Mattel introduced "Growing Up Skipper," a doll that grew breasts when you pushed back her arms. For once, little girls got a chance to control the uncontrollable. This Skipper came with two changes of clothes—a little girl outfit for the prepubescent look, and sophisticated eveningwear for the busty little doll.

We know that Barbie is just a doll—her proportions don't

match those of real women. But little girls love her. (Mattel estimates that somewhere in the world every second they sell two Barbies.) "I had that Barbie doll image tattooed on my brain," recalled thirty-three-year-old Cassie, now a writing professor. "I wasn't allowed to play with Barbie at home since Mom was a nurse and thought that Barbie was a gross misrepresentation of female anatomy. I was given Midge, a flat-chested, freckled, girl-next-door kind of doll. I disliked Midge intensely because she wasn't at all curvy and sexy like Barbie."

Some girls modify their Barbies as they become aware of female anatomy. A friend of mine gave her Barbie pink nail polish nipples. And Carla, forty, stuck straight pins in her Barbie's chest and painted them red for a more realistic look. Cassie remembers asking her mother why her breasts weren't smooth like Barbie's. She was lectured about human anatomy and what breasts are for: feeding children. "After that I felt a bit squeamish about breasts. Still, I thought Barbie was beautiful in all of her smoothness. To this day she affects me."

Often our first encounter with real non-Barbie breasts is seeing our mother or another woman breast feed. My first breast experience (after weaning) was watching my little brother get his turn at my mother's breast. I don't remember the specifics of it, although there's a photo of my mother breast feeding my brother while I'm standing to the side, looking on. "When I see a mommy breast feeding, I get very curious and I try to get a little peek," said six-year-old Ghyslaine who is fascinated by breasts, which she calls "baby bottles." Think about it. The idea of a woman putting her breast in a baby's mouth to feed that baby *is* amazing. There's no other body part that can work such magic.

As children we tend to assume that our mother's breasts are the norm. "Mommy has the biggest boobies!" says two-year-old Julia, who likes to "give boobie" to her stuffed animals. In fact, Julia's mother has small breasts, but these are the only breasts that Julia knows. Dylan, twenty-two, recalled: "When I saw a family friend in jeans and a bra, I suddenly realized how *huge* my mom's breasts were compared to her friend's, which were about a 34C, like mine now." Dallas saw the everyday breasts of the women around her as being much less desirable than her fantasy "Boob Shaker" breasts. "I felt a little sorry for these women with giant balloons strapped to their bodies."

Other women shared memories of breasts symbolizing comfort, love, and warmth. "My grandmother was telling me a story and I put my head on her shoulder and fell asleep cupping her breasts," remembered thirty-year-old Nia. "It just felt so comfortable and natural to do that. That's the closest I've ever been to her."

Learning that breasts are private is an important lesson. Andrea, thirty-three, discovered this when she was six and her twelve-year-old sister was starting to develop breasts. "I went into the bathroom while she was in the tub and I gave her boobs a poke because they fascinated me—they were so round and buoyant in the water. She said, 'Don't do that! They're private property.' I always remembered that." Thirty-two-year-old Sandra, who is Korean American, was raised by her parents to be very modest. "My little sister and I were both Campfire Girls. We were hiking once, and the two group leaders took off their tops. My sister and I were stunned. I just stared at these two women, thinking 'They are naked.' Not only that, but they each had very different breasts. The brunette had big breasts and dark nipples. And the other one, a redhead, had very fair skin and even whiter boobs, with very pink nipples."

As soon as we learn that breasts are private, we set out to explore this new territory. Growing up in Idaho, Carla carefully studied her parents' *National Geographic* magazines to get a glimpse of naked breasts, which she then sketched in hiding. She made hundreds of drawings, which she later burned to destroy the evidence. Scarlett, forty, remembered a slightly older girl from her Long Island neighborhood: "She asked me if I wanted to know what it was like being with a man. We both got undressed, and I lay on top and she had me touch her breasts. She had tiny breasts, but her nipples were erect and her skin was covered with goose bumps. We got dressed quickly when my mother came home, and this girl warned me not to tell anyone ever."

And we learn that breasts can be sexually attractive—even to us. Beth, twenty-five, remembered the first time she saw a woman's breasts: "I was ten and I was sleeping over at my friend's house. Her mom came in to kiss us good night, and as she leaned over I remember seeing her breasts and being aroused and fascinated by them, and then being really aware of what I was thinking. I'm sure I blushed."

As little girls, we may fantasize about growing breasts, but the reality may be complicated. Margie, thirty-six, dreamed of growing a huge pair of breasts like her grandmother's. "My cousin convinced me that the secret to Grandma's bosom was cold cream, and if I applied this miracle cream, I too would blossom." It didn't work—Margie now has small A-cup breasts. Leigh, twenty-three, associated having breasts with being grown-up: "Whenever I threw a penny into a fountain, looked up at the stars, or had a birthday, I wished for breasts, and braces." Before puberty, Marie, now twenty-nine, used to pester her mom: "When am I gonna get breasts?" She thought it would be fun to pretend she was a stripper, to dance and undress herself in front of a mirror. "Then, around ten, when my breasts started growing, I didn't want them anymore."

Nine-and-a-half-year-old Ali started developing at age seven, and has worn a bra ever since then. Now a 34B, she has slightly larger breasts than her mother, Judith, who has "spent a lot of energy making her feel good about her breasts and helping her cope with the other girls making fun of her." Ali's favorite comeback for classmates' teasing is: "The women on TV paid a lot of money for what God gave me for *free!*" Ali's breasts unceremoniously shoved her out of the world of childhood and into puberty. "She's a beautiful girl who has the body of a fourteen or fifteen year old," says her mother.

Ali knows that she stands out among the other girls in her third grade class. "I hope more girls start developing next year, not just the chubby girls." She also complains about the pain of growing breasts: "Sometimes they get on my nerves. Whenever I bend down at school and hit the desk they *really* hurt. When I first started showing, I was happy until they started hurting. Like when I run. I would get mad and yell at myself, 'I wish they were never here!'" Ali tells a funny story that reminds me of my own childhood superstitions: "My best friend would rather have boobs first than last. I told her that I heard that lima beans would make your boobs grow, so she went home and ate two cans of lima beans after school. She said she was about ready to puke afterwards."

While Judith teaches her daughter that she's "more than a cup size," Ali gets many messages to the contrary. Ali reasons that, "Just because girls have boobies on their chest, they don't have to show them to the world." And she's concerned that women use their breasts to get attention. Among her peers, she notes that girls seem more interested in breasts than boys do. "I guess girls want to have big boobs so they can look like TV stars." But despite all the difficulties of her early development, when asked if she'd rather have breasts or not, Ali ponders this and decides that she'll keep her breasts after all.

These stories aren't just child's play—they set the stage for our individual breast stories. These early experiences have important ramifications that surface again and again in each new phase of our lives: during puberty, motherhood, and our later years; in shaping our sexuality and our identity; and in our attitudes about health issues. This book continues and expands the dialogue that began in *Breasts*, the documentary. Whether you're a grown woman who wishes that breasts had been more openly discussed during childhood, a mother who can begin a new dialogue with her daughter, or a girl who is approaching these issues for the first time, I encourage you to start your own conversation about breasts. It's a simple yet radical idea—women talking honestly with other women about their breasts—and it can begin in the earliest years.

apples, babaloos, bags, bazongas, bazooms, Berthas, big brown eyes, blubbers, bobbers, boobies, boobs, bosoms, boulders, brace and bits, breast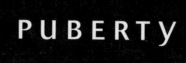s, buffers, b ssabas, cat a arlies, charms, chest, chestnuts, cliff, coconuts, cups, dairies, diddies, dinners, doorknobs, droopers, dumplings, eyes, fried eggs, gazombas, globes, gondolas, grapefruits, ha has, Harry and Junes, headlights, hooters, ice cream scoops, jersey-cities, jugs, kajoobies, knobs, knockers, lemons, love pillows, lungs, mammae, mammary glands, maracas, marshmallow mountains, melons, milk bottles, milkers, mosquito bites, nice ones, nipples, nips, orbs, pair, pancakes, peaches, pumps, puppies with the pink noses, rack, second pair of eyes, snack trays, sweater meat, ta tas, teats, the girls, tits, titties, tomatoes, torpedoes, twins, udders, upper frontal superstructure, walnuts, water balloons, watermelons, whales

"Are you there God? It's me, Margaret. I just told my mother I want a bra. Please help me grow God. You know where. *I want to be like everyone else."*

—Judy Blume
   Are You There God? It's Me Margaret[1]

When I was ten I started to keep a diary. Next to obsessing endlessly about crushes on boys and ups and downs with friends, I complained about how slowly my body was changing. In three separate dates, my careful measurements charted my breast growth: April 25, 1980: 26 inches; June 20, 1980: 26 1/4 inches; April 27, 1981: 27 3/4 inches. "Or more" was my hopeful addition. *I was a freak! Smaller than any girl ever!* I cheated when I measured myself, inhaling to widen my chest, and holding the measuring tape as loosely as possible. In a 1964 article in *Seventeen*, girls are told that ideally the bust should be ten inches larger than the waist, though a variation of an inch or two might be tolerated.[2] In my case, my body had three nearly equal measurements: breasts, waist, and hips.

Puberty is a crisis, wrote Simone de Beauvoir in *The Second Sex* in 1949. All of the internal mental and emotional upheaval of puberty is mirrored in the literal upheaval of our bodies; we look different and everyone in our lives—our family, friends, boys—starts looking at us differently. Simone de Beauvoir said that the developing girl's body is no longer "the straightforward expression of her individuality; it becomes foreign to her; and at the same time she becomes for others a thing: on the street men follow her with their eyes and comment on her anatomy."[3]

Although our first period is an important part of puberty, it is invisible to the outside world. Breasts are a public rite of passage, a sign on your chest that announces, "I am a sexual being." "You feel like you're not a child anymore," explained thirteen-year-old Teresa. "When you start developing breasts, you're treated more like a grown-up." But development is also an intensely private experience that can be alternately mysterious, scary, and exciting. Too often the lack of honest dialogue about this process can lead to serious misunderstandings. Many women confessed they thought they had breast cancer when they first felt their painful and hard breast buds. The rare girl who experiences development as positive does so because her family is open and honest.

Dr. Tian Dayton, a New York-based clinical psychologist who works with adults and teens, is the mother of a son and daughter, and describes this time as a phase where adolescent girls "don't know what's going to happen next." As children, we achieved a kind of androgyny, but developing breasts put an end to that period. This is the age at which girls feel pressure to stop being tomboys—if not overtly, then in many subtle ways. So while some girls seem to welcome a more womanly body, not surprisingly, many experience breasts as limiting. For Beth, twenty-five, the change was dramatic: "One day when I was twelve, I was walking home from soccer practice and a guy drove by and yelled something about my boobs. I had been ignoring that I had breasts, but it hit me then that other people saw me as a woman. That's the last time I played sports until I was in college. I decided that if I pretended I didn't have a body, then it wasn't there."

At puberty, our breasts change in size and shape under the influence of estrogen and progesterone, the two hormones that control menstruation. The ovaries start to secrete estrogen, which adds fat to the breasts, making them larger. Sensitivity to estrogen and progesterone varies from one woman to the next and determines the ultimate size of our breasts. The more sensitive the hormone receptors are, the larger the breasts. But no matter how or when we develop, there's so little dialogue about the experience that nearly every girl has a warped sense of her own breasts. The complaint "I didn't fit in" is voiced again and again.

How comfortable we are with this transition depends on how soon we develop and how others react to us. Love them or hate them, we construct our self-image in response to our breasts. And puberty is where it all begins. We compensate for our breasts, show them off, or play them down. Suddenly, we're pushed into competition with other girls and adult women—and all of this is beyond an adolescent girl's control.

For some teenaged girls, shame complicates this already difficult phase. Not only are our bodies changing faster than we can come to terms with, this public change attracts more attention than we may be able to handle. Unfortunately, during puberty negative attention is a common reality. While this may range from verbal harassment to sexual abuse, the problem worsens when girls are unable to confide in an adult and blame themselves. "If I didn't look like this, this wouldn't have happened," twenty-five-year-old Mona recalled thinking after one incident in fifth grade. Of course, looks have little to do with this—girls of all shapes and sizes have to deal with unwelcome attention.

The new focus on our breasts brings conflicted feelings of pleasure and guilt. Many girls try to disguise newly swelling breasts by wearing baggy shirts and oversized sweaters. Others experiment with their newfound power and test limits by dressing provocatively. For Carol, twenty-one, showing off cleavage was a way of not disappearing. As one of the few Latina students in an affluent and predominantly white private school, she was often overlooked because she couldn't compete with the other girls who could afford expensive clothes, stereo systems, and even cars. But she could compete with her body because "when guys see breasts they're gonna look."

Where do girls learn what *real* breasts look like? Like most girls, I had few realistic images against which I could judge my breasts. Television, movies, magazines, and nippleless Barbie provided a steady diet of unreal breasts. Women remembered Charlie's Angels running around braless, jiggling while chasing down bad guys; the cartoonish Barbara Eden in *I Dream of Jeannie*; or Betty and Veronica, actual comic book characters. Even young girls featured in animated Disney films are portrayed as having full breasts. It's no wonder we were confused. Sandra, thirty-two, recalled that it wasn't until a junior high gym class that she realized that girls' bodies looked different from each other. Briar, twenty-two, and her best friend, Melissa, had their own way of sizing themselves up. Briar remembered that they would "stand in front of the mirror with our tops off and talk about what was good or bad about our breasts."

While dialogue between friends helps, honesty is sometimes difficult to come by. Jill and Morgan, both in the seventh grade, were nonchalant about this phase of their lives, but their constant assertion that "we don't care about breasts!" wasn't terribly convincing. There was much eye-rolling as I asked them about breasts, bras, and boys. *Long sigh, giggle.* "You grow them and then you have them for the rest of your life. It's not like you're jumping out of a window and into the street!" said Morgan. They said that in their Manhattan school, "no way would you not wear a bra." Things heated up when Morgan accused Jill of not wearing a bra. Jill denied this vehemently, then admitted that she was wearing an undershirt. "It's true!" Morgan cried triumphantly, "She doesn't have anything to jiggle, she's so flat-chested!" Jill blushed and glared, "So?" So, Jill and Morgan care about breasts after all.

Our Mothers

"Luckily my mother's attitude was always positive, never ashamed, embarrassed, or teasing."

—Carmen, twenty-nine

Puberty is the moment when we start to look like and identify with our mothers, even as we are trying to forge our own identity. How a mother feels about her breasts, her degree of modesty, and how she talks to her daughter about developing all help determine how a pubescent girl feels about her breasts. Mothers may be threatened by their daughters' youth and emerging sexuality or they may celebrate it—and this can make a big difference in how their daughters see themselves. I grew up with open and supportive relationships with both of my parents, but strangely enough, breasts seemed to be an off-limits topic of discussion. It was easy to talk about menstruation, we had a celebratory dinner for my first period, but I don't remember ever talking with my mother specifically about breasts. I'm not sure why since my parents weren't puritanical about their bodies.

Whether or not we look like our mothers, many of us

measure our breasts against theirs. I sometimes saw my mother's breasts—"real" C-cup breasts that had nursed two children, with dark, round areolae and nipples that stuck out, unlike my flat, pale nipples. I always thought mine would look like hers someday, but I wound up with a very average-sized B-cup. As much as she wanted to grow up, twenty-two-year-old Dylan was intimidated by her mother's large breasts, which Dylan described as "3,460 double D-cup." Thirty-three-year-old Cassie was "horrified and fascinated by the incredible stretch marks from breast feeding" on her mother's breasts and hoped that she wouldn't get breasts like hers. And Sandra, a thirty-two-year-old first generation Korean American, grew up with parents who were extremely modest about their bodies. She remembered feeling guilty when she saw her mother's breasts: "I was curious about the way they looked, but I also felt bad because it was dirty to stare at your mother's breasts."

Some adolescent girls face puberty without a mother. Whether that absence is because of death or separation, it makes this phase much more difficult. When Sarah was in junior high, not only did she have to cope with the hassles of being an early developer, she was also in the process of losing her mother, who died of breast cancer when Sarah was only twelve. Now fifty, Sarah recalled that she didn't consciously make the connection between the location of her mother's illness and her own breasts, which she described as "out-of-control." Other women who lost their mothers to breast cancer at an early age remember feeling terribly conflicted and afraid of their own breasts for years after. Karin, a twenty-nine-year-old novelist and health educator, lost her mother to breast cancer when Karin was twenty. For years, Karin associated breasts with her mother's death, which made it virtually impossible for her to feel sexual pleasure in her breasts.

Mothers can also help clarify the many mysteries of puberty. Thirteen-year-old Teresa was worried that something was wrong when she felt pain as her breasts were developing, but her mother's clear explanation about the process comforted her. Teresa lives in a household that includes her parents, her aunt and uncle, and four kids. Her mother and her Aunt Lisha have had a frank, but playful, attitude throughout Teresa's adolescence, and it's clear that this positive reinforcement has helped Teresa. "My mom and I can talk about anything, so I wasn't embarrassed to talk to her about developing. Now she'll tease me sometimes, to make me laugh. She might say, 'Tie those things down, you might poke somebody's eye out!'" The lighthearted teasing and joking is a way of keeping perspective about her changing body, and it seems to work for Teresa. For Carmen, twenty-nine, the frustration of being small-breasted was tempered by her awareness that her mother and her older sisters had also been slow developers. "We all knew how difficult it was to wait and feel inferior. Luckily my mother's attitude was always positive, never ashamed, embarrassed, or teasing."

Harriet, fifty-six, wasn't as fortunate. Her mother shamed her for being small-breasted. "I started out and ended up with AA-cup breasts. My mother was always concerned about marrying me off—preferably to a rich man. I'm plain-looking— nothing spectacular—and my looks and small breasts weren't good enough for her." Whether it's boys, clothing, or makeup, fighting with our mothers is such a hallmark of growing up, it sometimes seems as if it's a pubescent prerequisite. But as much as teenage girls struggle to be independent, this is also the time when they most need support and encouragement from their mothers.

The First Bra

"I wanted everyone to know I had a bra and was becoming a woman."

—Lucille, seventy-six

In seventh grade I asked my mother to take me bra shopping, even though I was barely beginning to develop. I asked in the car—a clever move to minimize eye contact. I was so embarrassed, I might as well have been telling her that I wanted to dance in a nudie bar. "Why?" was her logical but devastating response. I didn't ask again. That year, I got a hand-me-down bra—ironically, from a younger friend. It was just a few elastic straps and two little white stretchy polyester-cotton triangles, with, of course, a pink bow in the middle. After a couple of extremely uncomfortable days, I stopped wearing the bra.

For most girls the first bra is a training bra. It serves less to support a girl's breasts than to support her sense of growing up. After all, bra equals woman. Every part of it is adult—the straps, the complicated hooks, the fabric, the colors. Teresa, thirteen, defined training bras as being for "people whose breasts are in training." When we put on that first training bra, we *are* in training for what it's going to be like to wear a bra, to have breasts, to be a woman. When Teresa tried on her first bra, she realized that it was the beginning of a whole new phase of her life: "I felt like I was growing up, and I felt so weird because it was a first-time thing. Now that I'm a teenager and getting closer to being able to get pregnant, I just want to take it slow."

Every year the drama of the first bra is played out in cities and towns all over America. Millions of girls and their mothers go through the initiation rite that millions of mothers and daughters have experienced before them. The whole activity of bra shopping is fraught with meaning. ("It's *not* like shoe shopping," explained Teresa.) Many women remembered feeling humiliated and embarrassed as they watched their mothers casually browse through the bra section in their local department store, touching the bras, asking questions. "I wanted to die," recalled Leigh, twenty-three. "I freaked out and we had to leave without buying anything."

Not all parents understand the significance of the first bra. Thirty-three-year-old Cassie, who was small-breasted, was desperately eager for a bra when she was eleven. Under five feet tall and barely over sixty pounds, she went on strike, refusing to wash or comb her hair until her mother took her bra shopping. "I insisted on wearing that bra all the time, even though it was maddeningly itchy and too big all the way around. The straps would slip off my shoulders and hang down on my bare arms. My father used to tease me about it: 'Cassie, you better pull up your bra strap, you don't want to have sagging breasts.' This was the big joke on one family vacation—me and my sagging breasts."

Some girls are forced into wearing bras before they are mentally or emotionally ready—even if their breasts might seem ready. Beth, twenty-five, felt that her body was out of control and "was freaked out at the prospect of having a woman's body." Her mother had to "drag" her to the department store to buy a bra, remind her to wear it, and tell her when it was getting too small. "I was really upset when I grew out of my bras. I wore bras that were too small for ages because I just didn't want to deal with it." Twenty-four-year-old Carrie wasn't able to tell her mother how afraid she was to be the first sixth grader in her school to wear a bra. Instead, fearing that her classmates would label her a "slut" because of her new bra, Carrie would wear the bra to school, take it off in the bathroom, and hide it in her book bag. Before she went home at the end of the day, she would put it back on so her mother wouldn't know.

Not all the pressure to wear a bra comes from mothers. Vicky, thirty, described herself as having had "*no* boobs at all" during puberty. She had large nipples, but little actual breast fat. Neither she nor her mother felt any need to buy her a bra until a teacher pulled Vicky aside, and told her that "it would be a good idea" if she started wearing a bra, presumably to disguise her nipples. "This was a big shock to me, and I remembered feeling embarrassed and ashamed about it afterwards. It felt like a direct, pointed statement toward my 'inadequacy.'"

For twenty-nine-year-old Leslie, the pressure to wear a bra also came at school. In her case, it was fear of humiliation brought on when her seventh grade class was being screened for scoliosis, and the girls were told that they'd be examined *topless* in front of their female classmates. Even though it was just a rumor, Leslie wore heavy sweaters for the rest of the year (even on the hottest days) to disguise her bralessness. That year, an old training bra came to her in a box of hand-me-down clothes from a cousin. Leslie remembered feeling "ecstatic, fascinated, scared, and ashamed all at the same time." Still, her first bra was contraband to be hidden away at all costs. She continued to wear her heavy sweater, now to disguise the fact that she *was* wearing a bra. She ended up abandoning the bra after a year, and now a 34A, she's happy to be braless.

Not all first bra experiences are so fraught with anxiety. Lucille, seventy-six, was thrilled by her first bra, which was a hand-me-down from a cousin. "I wanted everyone to know I had a bra and was becoming a woman, so I kept adjusting the straps and fiddling with the bra. I couldn't talk to my mother about it; she was foreign born and you just didn't talk about that sort of thing."

I bought my first real bras after my first year of college. At my mother's suggestion, we drove nearly two hours to the nearest mall where she got me two underwire bras (one black, one pink) and one cream-colored soft cup that was quite similar to my very first training bra. It was great fun picking out the bras and trying them on—pure celebration, no embarrassment. I'd wish this for every girl buying her first bra—the catch is, of course, that I was eighteen years old.

Our Fathers

Even if we see still ourselves as girls, our fathers begin to recognize us as women.

Puberty complicates the father/daughter relationship. Breasts literally and figuratively come between us. Some women stopped hugging their fathers as much when they developed breasts. One young woman said that the feel of her breasts pressing against her father's chest felt "too sexual" and that, though they never spoke about it, their hugs eventually evolved into a less intimate pat on the back. "I was no longer a child," said Annie, twenty-five. "I wasn't Daddy's sexually neutral little girl anymore. I was in on the secret—I had breasts, breasts equal sex, and sex was bad, so somehow I was bad now, too."

Even if we still see ourselves as girls, our fathers begin to recognize us as women. Lorraine, forty-nine, said that as a teenager she had regular run-ins with her father because of her penchant for tight sweaters. She recalls that at the time she feared that the stress of their conflict had a physiological impact on her hormones, which caused her to develop more slowly. Carol, twenty-one, found her father's protective reaction to her early development difficult to cope with. In the summertime in her Bronx neighborhood, kids stayed cool in the water at the fire hydrant. But the summer after third grade, Carol's father forbade her to play in the water because he worried that the neighborhood boys and men would ogle her. She watched her brother and all her friends from the window and felt "terribly excluded." Nia, thirty, grew up in a household where both parents and children were comfortable being nude or in their underwear in front of each other. But at age twelve, after a summer vacation spent away from home, her father's attitude changed. "While everyone was in my bedroom looking at pictures, I stripped down to my bra and underwear and my father said, 'Nia.' I didn't know what he meant until he said, 'You're getting older now, put your robe on.' And then it hit me that it was because I now had breasts."

Anna, twenty, always had a close relationship with her father as a girl. But at puberty, when she developed extremely large breasts seemingly overnight, their relationship changed. Her 34E breasts attracted a lot of attention at school and one day, after a particularly difficult encounter with some older high school boys, she went to her father for comfort. "I was upset, and he sort of laughed it off, saying, 'Boys will be boys.'

I was furious and hurt—how dare he brush off my humiliation and excuse them? This was *my dad* who had understood everything up to this point. I lost faith in him that day and I saw that he was just like them." Later, when she was sixteen, she had breast reduction surgery, a decision both her parents supported.

Zoe, twenty-five, grew up with a mother and stepfather who were open about sex and with whom she felt comfortable talking about the changes in her body. She was excited by the first signs of development when her nipples became what she called "puffy." However, her stepfather teased her, calling them "puppy" nipples. "That year for my birthday, my stepfather made a joke bra out of Dixie cups and string and gave it to me in front of everyone. His teasing was humiliating and it taught me a shame about my body that I hadn't experienced previously."

It's hard to say what our fathers could do to support us during puberty—talking openly about breasts seems next to impossible. I told my dad when I got my period, but I didn't talk about breasts with him, that seemed more intimate somehow. Although Ann, fifty, developed full breasts at age ten, the moral support of both her mother and her father helped her feel more excited and proud about having breasts. Breasts have a necessary though uncomfortable function in the father/daughter relationship. They shove us off his lap—the fact is, as teenagers we aren't Daddy's little girl anymore. So as difficult as this passage can be for both father and daughter, it's a transition that must take place.

Early and Late Bloomers

The lament, "I'm not normal!" is all too normal.

Almost every adolescent girl thinks of her developing breasts as too big or too small, too fast or too slow. I used to stand in front of the mirror studying my profile, wishing for breasts big enough to lift the fabric of my shirt away from my chest. I'd compare myself to the smiling girls with perfect breasts in the breast development chart in *Changing Bodies, Changing Lives*. I truly believed that I'd be happier and more attractive if only I had bigger breasts. I watched my best friend from eighth grade become popular when she ditched her thick glasses and showed up with *boobs* in ninth grade.

Of course, there is no *right* size—it all comes from the messages adolescent girls are receiving. And so many of those messages have to do with what's in vogue at the moment. Helene, eighty-seven, came of age during the tail end of the flapper era when the flat chest was in. "Girls with swelling breasts were regarded as somewhat *fast*, and the moment the breasts began to appear, we all wore the tightest bras that we could find." Fifty-nine-year-old Lynn, who was a 32A in high school thirty years after Helene, dreamed of being like Marilyn Monroe and Jane Mansfield, the sex goddesses of her youth when a big bust and a skinny waist were the rage. Mary, forty-eight, and a D-cup in junior high, came of age in the '60s when *Seventeen* magazine featured skinny Twiggy-type models. So, contrary to Lynn, she fantasized about a fairy that would transform her large breasts into "just normal sized—*maybe a little bit big.*"

The language may have changed over the years, but the message is the same. Countless teen magazine articles reassure readers that we come in all different shapes and sizes, then describe how we can be more like the *right* shape and size. They exhort teens to "minimize that ample bust" or dress up a flat chest with light padding or ruffles. The lament, "I'm not normal!" is all too normal. Teen magazines are packed with desperate letters: "My breasts are lopsided!" "My nipples look weird!" "I'm totally flat-chested!" "I'm too busty, everyone thinks I'm a slut!"

Products like the Mark Eden Bust Developer were a success precisely because of these insecurities. The Bust Developer was a pink plastic, spring-loaded device that fit in the palms of both hands. By pushing the two sides together between your palms, your chest muscles got a workout. The advertisements in the back of women's magazines claimed that women who used the Bust Developer often went from an A-cup to a D or DD. Gennifer, forty-eight, paid $9.98 for her Bust Developer in 1963 when she was thirteen. "I don't know if it worked or not because two days after it arrived, it mysteriously disappeared. I believe my parents had something to do with that."

Whether or not the definitions of early and late development are helpful or accurate, these terms are all too real to adolescent girls. Dr. Jeanne Brooks-Gunn, a professor of child development and education at Columbia University, conducted the "Adolescent Study Program," and found that girls who develop breasts before age eleven experience three times the risk of depression, eating disorders, and behavioral problems as do "normal" developers during adolescence.[4] Mona and Sharon, both in their twenties, used food to control their changing bodies. Mona reacted to the attention she received in fifth grade by putting on weight: "I wanted to look like I was flat from my breasts down." She thought that if she developed a big enough stomach, she would achieve her desired look. Sharon, on the other hand, starved herself for years. "I was afraid of growing up, and growing breasts was proof that it was going on, whether I liked it or not. My lowest weight was eighty-six pounds. My breasts shrank and I lost all the weight I gained throughout puberty, and then some." Sharon received treatment for anorexia, and still works hard to accept her body as it is.

Girls who develop earlier than their peers must cope with teasing and envy. Lisha, thirty-three, started growing breasts at the age of eight, and was wearing bras before any of the girls in her class. "From age ten through my teen years, it was horrible. I cried all the time. I was like a novelty that everybody picked on in school. They followed me around, and snapped my bra. By the time I was in fifth grade, I was 5'8" and a 34C, and that was too much. No one spoke to me, and when people did, they spoke to my chest. I hated my breasts and wanted to hide them. It wasn't until I got much older that I finally came to grips with them."

Many girls feel conflicted about the attention they receive for their breasts. "I thought that it was my fault that I had large breasts and that I was getting this attention," said Mona, twenty-five. "It took me years to understand that I had no control over it. I remember being ten and on vacation, walking with my mom and my grandmother down the boardwalk at Venice Beach, and this man looked me up and down and said, 'Ooh baby, nice tits!' I was just a *little girl* still watching the *Smurfs* on Saturday morning, but looking more like I was fifteen—I felt more vulnerable at that moment than I had ever felt in my entire life." Miriam, thirty-seven, started developing at age ten, and by thirteen had a full C-cup. Two years later, they increased to a D-cup. "I had the body of a woman, but I was a girl. People assumed that I should be more mature and sexually precocious because I looked it. I was both aware and titillated by the power I had, but also sort of embarrassed by it. By the time I was fourteen or fifteen I really shut down in the body department."

One of the risks for early developers, Dr. Brooks-Gunn found, stems from the girls' tendency to hang out with older teenagers who are already experimenting with sex. Adults, she added, are likely to treat these girls as if they are more mature. "We need to help folks realize that your developing nine-year-old is still a nine-year-old. The trick is supervision and monitoring. They can't stay out late just because they look older."[5]

Some parents try to warn their daughters about the harm that could come to them from unscrupulous boys, but inadvertently send the wrong message—that the girl is responsible because of her appearance. Marie, twenty-nine and an early developer at age ten, asked her mother what rape was after hearing a story on the local news. Her mother said that sex was a good thing when both people were in love and wanted to do it, but that sometimes boys forced girls to do it. Then she said boys were more likely to try that with girls who were more developed, like Marie was, so that was something she should watch out for. "I was already upset about my early blooming—this made my breasts an even bigger burden." During that entire year, Marie pinned her undershirts to her underwear, hoping to press her breasts flat against her chest. Mary, forty-eight, described her large breasts as a liability because of the constant attention. "It makes you distrustful of men, it makes you hate your body. It took actual trusting sexual experiences before my breasts really felt like they were me."

Many girls treat their large breasts as something alien to their bodies, to be denied and disguised. In high school, Carrie, now twenty-four, was labeled as "the girl with big tits." When she turned sixteen she dyed her hair pink and bright red because she didn't want anybody "to notice the rest of my body." Anna, who developed quickly to a 34E remembered, "I stopped wearing shirts that had anything written on them, because guys came up to me and drew their finger across the letters as if they were trying to sound out the word."

While girls with large breasts are shoved into the world of adults, late bloomers remain frozen in prepubescence. I remember thinking that without breasts, I didn't "have a body," as if I didn't exist. And then there is the constant teasing. In eighth grade, a boy I had a crush on insulted me with: "You remind me of a road from Dallas to Houston: no curves." (When I asked him about it years later, he swore that he had no memory of saying that.) But the negative comments don't just come from boys. Dallas, twenty-five, remembered seeing graffiti about her written by a girl in her junior high school locker room: "She's a carpenter's dream: flat as a board and never been nailed."

Some girls are able to turn the insults around and be more light hearted about being different. Janie, seventy-six, recalled, "I was flat-chested till I turned sixteen. I'd talk about it with my girlfriends, saying, 'I got marbles,' that sort of thing.

I resigned myself to the fact that I was flat-chested. And when prom time came, I filled up my bra with Kleenex. My mother found out, but she didn't say a thing. It just wasn't something you talked about. Not that I felt any shame about developing breasts, I just wished they'd hurry up and get there." Although Erika, twenty-eight, began developing at the same time as her peers, "everyone else kept on going and I stopped. It was hard for me. We were studying the Inuit Eskimos, so they called me Tundra, the flat lands." Erika and the other girls of the Tundra came up with a clever survival tactic. "In high school I was vice-president of the Itty-Bitty-Titty Committee. The president was my girlfriend who had smaller breasts than I did, but something strange happened to her when she went away to college and she hit a late puberty. When she came back, she had large breasts and we impeached her."

Birgitte, thirty, was a late developer, but when she bloomed she *really* bloomed. Now a voluptuous 38DD, she remembered: "All my girlfriends teased me that I had to fill my little bra with cotton or tissues because I had no breasts. It was an insecure point in my life. But all the women in my family had big breasts, so I knew I'd catch up. It was quite late, but I got the last laugh." The fact is, few of us feel that we developed right on time. The terms "early" and "late" developer are frustrating because they suggest that there's an exact time when we should sprout breasts. I love Erika's Itty-Bitty-Titty Committee and other girls' ways of coping with the early or late label. I propose throwing out those breast development charts—it's hard to find anyone who matches them anyway.

Second Base

"I knew, 'Ah, power. I have power with these things.'"

—Lynn, fifty-nine

Boys are desperately curious to know what is going on underneath girls' blouses. They communicate this in a variety of confusing ways: titty twisting, bra snapping, merciless teasing, annoying nicknames, or pursuing us openly, hoping to get a peek or a grope. "Boys adored my breasts, which was a blessing and a curse," remembered Sarah, a fifty-year-old teacher. Around this age, we may have been pleased by the attention from boys—but the overwhelming focus on our bodies, and particularly our breasts, could be less flattering.

At age thirteen, Teresa isn't romantically interested in

boys yet, but has noticed that the dynamic is changing: "No more, *'Cooties! Get away from me!'* You can tell the boys are really curious about us girls, but they don't talk about it in front of us. I'll walk by and hear them, and you know that's what they're talking about. I heard one boy say, 'I wonder what breasts are made out of.'"

Unlike some girls, Teresa is unwilling to accept any teasing. "If a boy comes up to me and says, 'Hey, Teresa's getting breasts,' I'm going to punch him dead in the face! But if they say that in my ear, and they're a close friend and they're only joking, I might say 'Hey' and push them or something, but not hard. I don't blame boys for noticing. They see that I'm growing up—I'm not the same old little Teresa anymore." Like Teresa, Beth, twenty-five, fought back against a boy who harassed her in junior high school. "He'd stand next to me and whisper and make comments about my breasts in a really immature but threatening way. I didn't tell anyone because I didn't want to draw any more attention to my body. Finally, one morning he asked me to come into a classroom down at the end of the hall because he wanted to see them. I went down the hall with him, and then smashed his head into the blackboard and slapped him across the face. He left me alone after that."

If most girls don't fight back, it's because they're too embarrassed or don't realize that they can stand up for themselves. Lynn, fifty-nine, remembered: "In high school the boys would come up to us when we were standing outside school, and stick their notebooks under our chests and say, 'Read this!' And if you could read the top lines, they would make fun of us, like our breasts were too small to cover the page. I was very offended, but we didn't know we were supposed to be feminists then, so we just let them do it. Besides, we wanted the attention." However, Scarlett, forty, didn't want the attention she got for her particularly large nipples—attention that made her feel self-conscious for years: "We were studying India, talking about the Taj Mahal. Somebody in the back of the class screamed out 'It's just like Scarlett's tits!' because of the little nipple-like thing on top. Everyone started calling me 'Taj' and the name stuck for a really long time. I started wearing padded bras just so you couldn't see my nipples. I even wore Band-Aids over them."

For girls whose friends include boys during childhood, there is often an abrupt change after their breasts start to develop. Lynn had been a tomboy, but the appearance of breasts ended her casual friendships with the neighborhood boys. "I used to tease them by standing by my window wearing a little strapless top and pulling it down so that they could see the top of my breasts, but not the nipples. I was a tease. It was terrible. I used to try and sex up these little twelve year olds. I guess I was aware it was naughty. I certainly never did it in front of my mother. But I knew, 'Ah, power. I have power with these things.'"

But even more than power, we discovered that we could have pleasure too. The same hormones that cause girls' breasts to swell also sensitize them, turning them into an erogenous zone. Most of us discovered this on our own before we ever let a boy anywhere near our breasts. Beyond exploring our own bodies, many of us experimented with girlfriends. Twenty-eight-year-old Valerie and her junior high girlfriends used to have wrestling matches—the main goal of which seemed to be to touch the other girls' bodies. "We never talked about it, and didn't recognize it as sexual, but looking back I think we were releasing some serious built-up sexual tension." And growing up in Idaho, forty-year-old Carla and her best friend would often spend the night at each other's house: "We would frequently wake up locked in a passionate embrace, aroused from kissing and fondling one another's breasts. All this was driven by dreams about boys we knew. We weren't quite sure what to do about it. She was afraid of being a lesbian, but overall I think we both liked it."

Sex during this time is mysterious, scary, and terrifically exciting. But unlike our adult years when touching, kissing, and sucking breasts is considered foreplay, during our teen years a little making out could go a long way. Breasts provide a safe and pleasurable way for teenage girls to explore their sexuality. And if sexual activity is limited to "second base," then breasts become that much more important to our sexual pleasure.

Part of sex as a teenager involves trying to find privacy. We made out in cars, friends' houses, movie theaters, parks— it was all so wonderfully illicit. I think of that time and remember holding my breath during those sessions with boys who, for the most part, were pretty clueless about what they were doing. I remember one particularly charming guy who, after kissing me and touching my breasts in the back seat of a friend's car, murmured in my ear, "Nice pecs."

Carol, twenty-one, recalled being with her eighth grade boyfriend in the dark of the back row of the local movie theater. "We were kissing, and then for the first time ever, he put his hand underneath my shirt and into my bra. Oh God, that was like fireworks going off. I don't think it's ever felt as good as the initial touch." Cecilia, thirty-one, described the classic baseball analogy of sex: "The game was—first base: kiss; second base: to get inside her shirt; third base: to get inside her pants; fourth base: to get inside her. I was good at this game and didn't lose my virginity until I went to college, but in junior high my friends and I played a game with some of the boys in drama club. If the girls wore a shirt with stripes, the boys would try to trace the stripes with their fingers as a way to get to touch our breasts (albeit through cloth). When I knew I'd be rehearsing with the boy I liked, I'd wear plaid, sit in his lap, and let him trace to his heart's content."

Teenagers come up with all sorts of games—all thinly veiled excuses for exploring sex. In my high school in Maine, the game was Truth or Dare. Girls wanted to kiss the cute guys and boys wanted the girls to take off their tops. The choice at that time seemed to be have breasts and get attention, or be flat-chested and get overlooked. Jean, thirty-one, who grew up in Manhattan, remembered playing Seven Minutes in Heaven in seventh grade. "I went out on the terrace with the boy who picked me for our seven minutes. It was a nightmare. I don't think I had any breasts at that time. I kissed him because that's what I had to do, and he put his hands up my shirt and started rubbing all over my chest. I screamed, ran to the freezer, grabbed a popsicle, put it down his shirt, and locked myself in the bathroom. I was so upset." Mona, twenty-five, remembered similar make-out parties in her junior high years. "It always felt really good when the guy's hand would go under my shirt. I was probably more in demand than the other girls—and that was fine with me. It felt really good to be wanted. We'd play Spin the Bottle or Three Minutes in the Closet, the lights would go out and people would partner off. For me, the rule was boys could touch me *only* above the waist. I really liked it, but I also kind of felt like I was going downhill on a roller coaster."

Ann, fifty, became aware of the potential of her breasts early on. "I was flirtatious and interested in the opposite sex as a kid. Not with intercourse, but with fooling around. When I was fourteen, I had a dream that my boyfriend lay on top of me touching my breasts and I had an orgasm. I knew immediately that my breasts were special, because they were so responsive and so happy to be touched." Later, Ann continued to have orgasms from breast stimulation.

With breasts come responsibility and power. Because

they are a public announcement of our coming of age, our breasts symbolize a loss of innocence and childhood. In a way, they don't belong to us anymore. They become a trophy to capture—they're currency in our relationships to everyone else. But it's a double-edged sword, because that power can turn against us. Were we "the girl with big tits" or the "nice girl" with small breasts? The constant comparison and yearning for normalcy begins here, and continues into our adult lives. We were in training, all right, but we desperately needed direction. And there are few of us who got the honest and direct guidance we needed.

apples, babaloos, bags, bazongas, bazooms, Berthas, big brown eyes, blubbers, bobbers, boobies,
boobs, bosoms, boulders, brace and bits,
breastices, Bristol City, bubs, buckets, buds, buffers, bumpers, bust, cans, cantaloupes, cassabas,
cat a   arlies,
char   cups,
daire   **IDENTITY**   opers,
dump   lobes,
gondolas, grapefruits, ha has, Harry and Junes,
headlights, hooters, ice cream scoops, jersey-
cities, jugs, kajoobies, knobs, knockers, lemons,
love pillows, lungs, mammae, mammary glands,
maracas, marshmallow mountains, melons, milk
bottles, milkers, mosquito bites, nice ones,
nipples, nips, orbs, pair, pancakes, peaches,
pumps, puppies with the pink noses, rack, second pair of eyes, snack trays, sweater meat, ta
tas, teats, the girls, tits, titties, tomatoes, torpedoes, twins, udders, upper frontal superstructure,
walnuts, water balloons, watermelons, whales

"And even now, now that I have been countlessly reassured that my figure is a good one, now that I am grown-up enough to understand that most of my feelings have very little to do with the reality of my shape, I am nonetheless obsessed by breasts. I cannot help it. . . . Well, what can I tell you? If I had had them, I would have been a completely different person. I honestly believe that."

—Nora Ephron
"A Few Words About Breasts"[1]

It should come as no surprise that our breasts have such a profound impact on our identity. Unlike any other part of our body, they are alternately hidden from view and shown off. They play an important role in all the areas of our lives: puberty, sexuality, motherhood, health, and aging. Our faces are our outward identity—our breasts are our public *and* private identity all in one. "I don't think we can talk about how a woman feels about her breasts in isolation," says Dr. Tian Dayton, an author and clinical psychologist in New York City. "I think it's always in relation to what the function of the breast is in her world, and that relates to men, to other women, to children." As women, many of us are accustomed to seeing ourselves in relation to others rather than as totally independent entities. We are mother, wife, lover, sister, daughter, friend, co-worker, and how other people react to us has a powerful effect.

Like Nora Ephron, I spent years hating my breasts. Having small breasts was an essential part of who I was—the way other people are tall or short, or of a specific race or nationality. Unlike most American girls, I never went on a diet and I didn't obsess about my weight. I didn't hate my nose or my hair. My breasts were the focus of my dissatisfaction: My tragic flaw was the fact that, as far as I was concerned, they didn't exist. I know that my life would've been radically different if I had had different breasts.

Growing up, I was younger than my classmates because I started school earlier than most kids. Had I been the same age as everyone else, I'm guessing that I wouldn't have seemed so far behind. I was small and thin—I didn't weigh above one hundred pounds until my second year of college. I was one of those girls who everyone described as "cute." I hated being cute. Cute doesn't mean sexy or beautiful, it doesn't mean *woman*—it means *little girl*.

In my world—a small public high school in Maine in the 1980s—breasts were a hot commodity, as was blonde hair, preferably long. I didn't have curves, plus I had short dark hair. But rather than blaming the standard of beauty, I came to dislike my breasts. My best friend at the time had full C-cup breasts and long blonde hair. She had boys lining up to go out with her, while I dated only occasionally. I'd quiz my male friends: Which do you prefer, big or small breasts? Most often they'd say that they didn't care, but I never believed them. If that was true, why were they chasing the girls with big breasts? After high school, none of my boyfriends ever complained about my breasts, but I still harbored the knowledge that I was deficient—*I must be lucky that they didn't notice.*

When I was twenty, I went to Paris to work as a nanny. I looked around and I seemed to fit the aesthetic, and being a young American woman in what I believed was the romance capital of the world didn't hurt. My body didn't change radically, but my attitude did. I still didn't need to wear a bra (I didn't wear one until I graduated from college), but suddenly my body was just right. My self-image and my body had gotten into sync. I was considered sexy and so I became sexy. Still, for a long time, it startled me to hear a man tell me that I had "perfect breasts."

The myth of the "normal" breast was finally shattered

for me when I began making the breasts documentary. Talking to hundreds of women and seeing so many real breasts made me feel better about mine—an experience that many viewers shared. Under the magnifying glass of this experience, my obsession crumbled. No longer the great and terrible Oz, it was a rather laughable worry. I finally realized that I'm not small—I'm medium. (One boyfriend even admitted to me that my breasts were a little "too big" for his taste.)

So what do my breasts really look like? They're a very round, medium-sized 34B (depending, of course, on the bra.) Like the rest of my complexion, they're pale and the left one has a small dark freckle. I used to dislike my nipples because they're light colored and don't stick out. Sometimes one gets hard while the other lies there passively. All in all, they're still pretty perky. So it was all in my head. For years I clung to my small-breasted identity because it was familiar. But today, I must admit, I'm rather fond of them.

I'm not recommending that everyone move to Paris or make a documentary film about breasts to feel better about their own. Some women have their own little epiphanies thrust on them, for others, it's a slow process of self-discovery. Regardless of the speed and magnitude of this process, I've realized that every woman has a story to tell about her breasts. More than just a story about a bra or an anecdote about puberty, these are stories of identity. How we view our breasts and, by extension, how we view ourselves, depends on a host of factors. The biggest question is, of course, are we satisfied with our breasts? What size are they, and how do we and others react to that? Do we show off or hide our breasts? Do we joke about them? Are we shy? What do we call them? Do we alter them surgically? What kind of bras do we wear? (Wonderbras? sexy ones? utilitarian ones?) Do we even wear a bra? How do we look at other women's breasts, and how do they look at ours? Do our breasts empower us or make us vulnerable? When it comes to breasts, there are no norms.

Love Them or Hate Them

*"I feel like I'm inadequate because I don't have 'perfect' breasts . . .
But I don't think I would change anything about my breasts,
because . . . I don't want to change anything about my body."*

—Molly, twenty-five

As women, finding fault with our bodies seems as natural
and predictable as breathing. We've been trained to do this—
and our breasts certainly don't escape the scrutiny. We judge
our nipples, the color of the areolae, the size of our breasts,
the amount of sag, stretch marks, and on and on. Gennifer,
forty-eight, a public relations specialist in the Midwest, has
undergone several cosmetic surgical procedures on her breasts.
"I've put 'the girls' and myself through a lot because of my
breast obsession. For my well being, I've come to realize it's
not my breasts that need changing, but my attitude about them,
and I'm working on that." Gennifer has worked hard to recon-
cile herself with her breasts—she even wrote a letter to them
to help sort out her feelings. "Is it possible to love you? I want
to, I know in my heart that I do. I have scrutinized you from
every angle, and on days when you appeared somewhat nor-

mal, I kept staring at you until I found something wrong. Only then would I look away, satisfied. Over the years, my hatred of you has taken on a mind of its own. It has become such a habit to despise you. It has taken so much energy from me."

However, Gennifer admitted to still wanting surgery: "I currently have implants, and intend to keep them. The issue I have now is one of symmetry—one breast has developed some scar tissue, the other hasn't. Someday when I have an extra $6,000 to fix them, I will do that, but for now, I'm satisfied with what I have. I look good dressed and okay undressed. At this stage in my life I am working harder at focusing on and appreciating my inner beauty than my outer beauty. After all, there is no end to the lengths we can go in order to measure up to the next woman, only to find there's *another* woman with bigger, perkier, softer, rounder breasts." While Gennifer tries to accept her body, it's clear that she is still cataloging what is wrong with her breasts.

Like Gennifer, Molly, twenty-five, is dissatisfied with her breasts, but decided not to get cosmetic surgery. Molly believes that her breasts, like the rest of her body, are who she is, and she's not willing to alter her self-image. "I feel like I'm inadequate because I don't have 'perfect' breasts," admitted

Molly. "They're floppy and saggy. They're so far from the norm—or what I have been raised to believe is the norm—that I'm kind of ashamed of them. But I don't think I would change anything about my breasts, because, on principle, I don't want to change anything about my body. I think I would like them to be a little firmer and perkier, but I don't, I don't."

Beyond what our breasts look like, there's also the matter of how they make us feel. How do they fit in with the rest of our personality? For Rhonda, twenty-three, her appreciation of her breasts is physical. She has coped with painful arthritis since early childhood and says, "My breasts are just about the only visible part of my body that isn't affected in some way by arthritis. They feel healthy and whole and complete, a feeling I don't have when it comes to my arms, legs, hands, feet, or hips. The fact that they are a part of me that the arthritis can't hurt makes me appreciate them more." Dallas, a twenty-five-year-old researcher, feels that her 34B breasts help her feel more "grown up" at times when she feels that she looks and feels "too young to be taken seriously."

A particularly telling example of breasts shaping a woman's identity is Racine, a tall, slim, flirtatious thirty-year-old who was working as a hostess in a fashionable New York

City restaurant when we first met. Since childhood, Racine had always dreamed of having breasts. "I was born a male, but mistakes are made." Unlike other women, Racine's breasts didn't develop naturally, so she treats them like a prize rose. Over the years she has had hormone treatments and several operations: "My breast story is interesting, because I know what it's like not to have any, then have small breasts, and now have larger breasts. It's been like the stock market, and now we're up and we're very bullish."

Racine was happy to lift her blouse to show me her full and natural looking breasts. At first glance, I didn't even notice the small scars around her areolae. She said she was proud of how men responded to them, and when she showed me to the door of the restaurant, a passing cab driver slowed down to ogle her, proving her point. Her breasts are important to her precisely because they, more than anything else, have shaped her public identity as a woman. "I think my breasts are absolutely the centerpiece of being a woman. When you see me standing here, all five feet, ten inches, my breasts speak for themselves. Even as a child I knew that having beautiful breasts, well-formed breasts, would get me all the attention and respect that I wanted. And I think they have. They get me through doors, in doors, out of doors, behind doors. I'm absolutely, one hundred and ten percent, positively in love with them."

Racine's power as a woman comes from truly claiming her breasts for herself. Power and vulnerability are two emotions that surface again and again when we talk about our breasts. Our breasts empower us when they send out a message that feels comfortable to us, but if we believe they're conveying the wrong message, they can make us feel defenseless. These feelings can change quickly depending on the circumstances. I can't imagine walking around wearing skimpy clothes like some women I've seen on the streets in New York. I don't like to be exposed to the comments and looks, and yet, at times, I love to show off a little, which can feel very powerful. Likewise, women share stories of being surprised by how powerful they felt going topless on a beach—where they felt safe to do so. Yet many of these women probably wouldn't feel comfortable going topless, or even showing too much cleavage, in another context.

Ilana, forty-seven, had a wonderful moment in her early twenties when allowing herself to be vulnerable with her breasts actually made her feel powerful. "In 1972 I was living in Berkeley, California with some male friends. One night it was really hot and humid and my roommates were all walking around in shorts and nothing else. Well, I was hot too, so I went into my room, took a deep breath, took off my shirt, and appeared in the kitchen with only my shorts on to help with dinner. I still remember the look of shock on their faces. I felt incredibly empowered." Marla, forty-four and the mother of three, draws strength from her breasts in a completely different way. "They make me feel powerful because these breasts grew three gorgeous children—solely on the milk that they produced. *That's power*."

While size may have something to do with the degree of power or vulnerability that we feel, as with everything, it's relative. Cassie, a thirty-three-year-old professor and a 34C, said that she feels "vulnerable because they make me feel marked. I rarely wear close-fitting clothes and I don't like people looking at my breasts. Usually, I wish I did not have them. They swing around and get in the way." Lisha, thirty-three and a 38FF, agrees. "I never felt power with them. I always felt that they controlled me more than I controlled them. I just never felt comfortable with them." However, Caroline, thirty-three and a 34B, said that since she's gone up a cup size this past year, "I feel stronger, like the female busts on the prow of a Viking galleon ship."

Whether or not we choose to show off our breasts is indicative of our feelings of power or vulnerability. Sandra, thirty-two and a 34B, recalled a time in her life when she had gained weight and was a C-cup. "Even with that one cup size difference, people looked at me differently. It made me sensitive. I guess I've been brought up to believe that if you dress sexy and show cleavage you're asking for it. It implies the wrong things to men." But Jean, thirty-one and a 36C, had a special New Year's resolution to overcome her habit of hiding her breasts. "I resolved to show more tit because I realized that I had these assets that I wasn't using. Whether it was just showing more tit or that I was psychologically unbuttoning myself, I suddenly got all the dates in the world."

While women like Jean have truly accepted their breasts as part of their identity, it's sad to see how many other women are dissociated from their bodies. Dr. Susan Love, a renowned breast surgeon, breast cancer expert, and mother of a ten-year-old daughter, believes that as women, we need to "reclaim our bodies. The process has started, but it's far from complete. Today, women are increasingly accepting their bodies in terms of reproduction and childbirth, but we still need to work on defining what our breasts mean and what their value is to us.

We can't let other people define our reality for us."[2] If we choose to define our own "breast reality," then making the move towards accepting and even loving our breasts—no matter what they look like—will be that much easier.

Measuring Up

"I find that I fantasize about having big breasts or about being someone different who has big breasts, but in reality, I like the way mine look."

—Charlotte, thirty-two

We're constantly being bombarded with conflicting messages about the "right" breast size. One month we're told that "big breasts are back." Three months later the same magazine will announce that a smaller, androgynous look is beautiful. In general, though, our society does tend to place more value on big breasts. Go through a day in our world—watch television, pick up a women's magazine, go to the movies, walk down the street. Guaranteed you'll see more big breasts than you'll know what to do with. Size matters. And it doesn't matter. Size is complicated because it can be connected to our identity in so many different ways.

The size and shape of our breasts can change with weight gain or loss, taking birth control pills, and pregnancy, among other things, but it's so public to the outside world that we tend to attribute certain personality traits to breast size, even if we should know better. We've all heard the hackneyed stereotypes about size—if you have small breasts, you've got to be serious, bookish, uptight, frigid. If you have big breasts, you must be oversexed, dumb, ditzy, easy, good in bed. Big breasts have become a punch line—look at the stock blonde with big boobs in any sitcom.

It's a stereotype Anne, fifty, has little patience with. As a 34D, she didn't let herself become branded simply as a big-breasted woman. Unlike some women, she refused to hide them away. Instead, she delighted in them, often wearing low-cut blouses. For her, being a sexy woman with big breasts didn't conflict in the least with being a highly competent, intelligent professional. "My mind and my body were totally integrated, and I had no problem conveying that to the world. I never had to explain to people that I was an intelligent woman—that came across in the first conversation. But I was also highly sexual. I saw no problem with being both."

The ideal breast size necessarily varies from one society to another, and even geography can play a big part in this. According to the American Society of Plastic and Reconstructive Surgeons (ASPRS), in 1992, nineteen percent of all breast augmentations were performed in California. Twelve percent were in Florida and ten percent in Texas.[3] Dr. Loren Eskenazi, a San Francisco-based plastic surgeon who specializes in breast surgery, said that anecdotally, the ideal in New York is more European, svelte, and androgynous. Most of the South and Los Angeles prefer bigger breasts.

Women who spend time in different cities around the country often experience varied attitudes depending on where they are. Charlotte, thirty-two and a 36B, lives in New York City, but sometimes works in Los Angeles in film and television, and is always struck by the difference between L.A. and New York breasts. "Everywhere you go in L.A. there are these Amazon women on billboards with giant implanted breasts and women standing in line at Starbucks in these microscopic bras with huge breast implants. It makes me feel defensive about my breasts. I find that I fantasize about having big breasts or about being someone different who has big breasts, but in reality, I like the way mine look. I think these huge implants look freakish and I think it would be horrible to have all the attention focused on something as dumb as your breasts."

Having lived in the Caribbean as well as various parts of the United States, Dallas, twenty-five and a 34B, has her own thesis on the link between society and breast size. "It seems to me that, in general, upper class people tend to prefer the smaller-breasted look. European and North American high fashion and haute couture enforce that with the androgynous small-breasted look, whereas working class men prefer the pin-up girl: buxom and curvy. I've come to notice small breasts with a degree of envy and large breasts with a degree of pity or repulsion."

Racial and ethnic groups also have their own stereotypes about size. Carol, a twenty-one-year-old student with 38DD breasts, was born in Puerto Rico and raised in New York City. "In the Puerto Rican culture, big breasts are definitely favored. With my family and friends, big breasts mean that you're more of a woman—good in bed, but also a good mother." Sandra, a thirty-two-year-old Korean American who works in advertising and has 34B breasts, complained, "I can't tell you how many guys have said, 'You've got big breasts for an Asian girl.' For a long time I thought it was true, too, and then finally I started looking around and noticed that it just wasn't so." And, according to Mary Ellen, a fifty-eight-year-old African American journalist with 36B breasts, "There's the sense that black men like women to have more body. They don't mind a woman with big breasts and a big butt. They don't like little skinny chicks."

Whatever attitudes we grew up with, we find different ways of integrating cultural biases with our own beliefs about breast size. As a teenager Harriet, fifty-six, felt terrorized about having 34AA breasts. Her mother equated being small-breasted with being an unsuitable wife. When Harriet went off to college in 1960 she found out that "nobody gave a shit about the size of my breasts. We were so intellectual. We sat around having discussions about Kant. In my whole life no one but my mother has ever been interested in my boobs. Certainly the man I married didn't care—he loved my breasts just the way they were."

Beth, twenty-five and a 38DD, changed her negative feelings about her big breasts, not with a reduction, but by adding a nipple ring. She heard friends rave about how it made them feel better about their breasts, but she hesitated because she wondered, "Do I really want to attract more attention to a body part I can just barely deal with as it is?" Finally she decided to take the plunge, and was more than pleased with the results.

"Since I got the piercing, my attitude has changed in so many ways. I show it to almost anyone I know who can deal with it. I can hardly believe it myself—I'm still uber-self-conscious around a lover, and here I am flashing my tits to people at work. I like the way it looks and I find it erotic and self-affirming at the same time. I think it's really my way of saying that I've spent more than a decade pretending I don't have boobs, and it's time to get over that and move on."

When I gathered a group of women together for a breasts discussion party, almost everyone who was small believed that big breasts were in, while the larger-breasted women honestly believed that small breasts were in vogue. So many of us seem to think that what other women have is better. While many smaller women have complicated stories, for larger-breasted women, the focus can be more intense, simply because their breasts are so obvious. But ultimately, size is relative. What may feel "huge" for one woman, might be "medium" for another. What's important is not the actual size of our breasts, but how we feel about them.

The AA to FF on Identity

"I found my bralessness was giving me a reputation so I had to bind them up again."

—Dallas, twenty-five

Bras, more than being simple undergarments, are another way of defining ourselves. From the little tag that classes bras from AA to FF, to the style of the bra, this sometimes flimsy, over-priced piece of underwear says a lot about who we are. We often describe women with their bra size—we'll even say that someone *is* a D-cup, not *has* a D-cup, as if a woman is her breasts. Briar, twenty-two, recalled two college friends who had a hard time accepting their cup sizes. "One was a big C and would squeeze into B bras because she didn't want to admit to being a C-cup. The other was a D and she was wearing C bras, because she complained that you couldn't find a sexy, pretty D bra. One day they finally decided to buy their correct bra sizes, and my D-cup friend gave all her C-cup bras to my C-cup friend and she went out to look for a nice bra. It was very freeing for both of them."

But bras are also about controlling our breasts, holding

them in. After all, the revolutionary act of women burning their bras in the late 1960s and '70s was a way of saying, "You can't hold us back or strap us down anymore." There's something threatening and powerful about a braless woman—too much jiggling makes people a little nervous. Dallas, twenty-five, recalled spending a summer in France where she went topless on the beach and stopped wearing a bra. "I lost much of my self-consciousness, but when I got back to the States, I found my bralessness was giving me a reputation so I had to bind them up again."

Leigh, twenty-three and a 36B, summed up what many women feel about bras: "I've asked myself if I would wear a bra if I lived only with women, in a huge house with lots of land, or on an island. I bet I wouldn't. My breasts aren't large enough that it makes a physical comfort difference. I wear one daily only because it makes a mental difference. Bras make me feel more secure and held in." Melissa, a twenty-seven-year-old research scientist who ranges between a 36A and B, complained about the stereotypical notion that women who don't wear bras are sluts. "I find myself thinking this sometimes and it makes me sick. Breasts jiggle, but we're so obsessed with strapping them down and making them more acceptable, not letting our nipples show through, forcing them into different shapes and positions. It's really sad that it's seen as unprofessional to be anything other than strapped down."

Finding the right bra can be far from fun. So many of us end up feeling frustrated and even lacking when we can't fit into the set sizes—and this applies to women with small, medium, and large breasts. Vicky, thirty-two, remembered her days as a 34AA before she got an augmentation. "When they did have a bra that fit it would always be padded with fiberfill, which is so insulting. If you look in the mail order lingerie catalogs you'll find that they don't have anything extraordinarily large or small that looks nice. If you fall outside of B, C, or D-cup, you have to go to a specialty shop like you're some sort of abnormal creature." Andrea, thirty-three and a 38C, described bra shopping as hell, because for a long time she could never find a pretty bra that would fit. "I used to get really upset. I'd always end up feeling ugly and non-sexy. My sisters would be wearing these really pretty, lacy little bras and I couldn't find anything that was attractive."

Louise, thirty-one, had her own dramatic bra-buying experience when she was shopping for a strapless bra for her wedding dress. A 38DD, Louise recalled, "I tried on every strapless bra in every department store. I couldn't find anything, and all these salesladies kept giving me these pitying looks and saying, 'I'm sorry dear,' like I was crazy to think that I could find a strapless bra. At one place, a saleslady pulled me aside and said, 'There's a store uptown. I used to do a little dancing myself.' She thought I was a hooker or an exotic dancer or something. I called the store and even they didn't have a strapless bra that would fit well. I came home practically in tears, and my mother sent me to Livi's Corsets, and Livia was there and she handed me a Goddess Bra in white. And my wedding was saved."

Livi's Corsets on the Upper East Side of Manhattan is owned and run by Livia Finger, at ninety, the oldest working brassiere saleslady in New York City. Since 1948, Livia has been making and selling brassieres, girdles, and corsets. Livia was born in Budapest, and came to New York in 1944, and she still hasn't lost her accent or her enthusiasm for lingerie. "There is nobody who has more experience. I can fit anybody, *dahling*. I have a lot of faithful customers. They always come to me and they don't let anybody fit them but me." Livia has particular ideas about the right look for bras: "Everything in good taste, *dahling*. You can have a push-up, but you have to look at the figure, waistline, and height of the person. That's where I come in and advise the customer. But you have to take the customer's wishes fifty percent, and I think I am usually the winner."

It's easy to be caught in a bra trap, a prisoner of elastic, lace, and cup size. But like the rest of our breast story, if we can keep the importance of bras in perspective, we might be able to avoid the tears, the frustration, and the sense of inadequacy at not being able to find a bra that fits well and looks good. Recently, Virginia Morton, a clothing designer, conducted an extensive study in which she measured over ten thousand women and came up with a whole new sizing system—with over one hundred and fifty different bra sizes. I guess it took a woman to come up with a new and saner way of recognizing that women—of all different shapes and sizes—can't be strapped down into a few inadequate cup sizes.

Downsizing

"One cup from my old bra could fit over my entire face."

—Nell, twenty-three

According to the American Society of Plastic and Reconstructive Surgeons (ASPRS), the number of breast reduction procedures increased from 39,639 in 1992 to 64,620 in 1997, at an average cost of $4,877.[4] Breast reduction—unlike augmentations or breast lifts—is a cosmetic surgery that our culture forgives. Because of our persistent stereotypes about size, many people respect women who get a reduction. It's as if by reducing her breasts, she's upping her intelligence quotient. Still, there are others, both men and women, who are surprised that a woman with large—and hence better—breasts would voluntarily make them smaller.

Today, as technology improves, there are fewer risks associated with breast reduction surgery. Loss of sensation is still a potential side effect, but the large scars of years past are less common. Dr. Eskenazi explains that there are often very real physical benefits that outweigh the risks, "There are people for whom the neck and back pain is intense. The average big reduction is about five to eight pounds of tissue. And if you took five to eight pounds and wore it on a string around your neck all day, you'd have back pain." Many of these women claim to feel empowered by shedding the literal and figurative burden of large breasts. I remember being surprised when three of my friends decided to have reductions. In my frame of mind, it seemed odd that they were willing to undergo surgery, and have permanent scars and loss of sensation, just to have smaller breasts. And yet, despite any of the physical drawbacks of surgery, most women are glad that they made the choice.

Three years ago, I got a call from Cindy who had read an article about the breasts documentary in a magazine. She was eager to speak to me because she had been considering a breast reduction and wanted advice. She'd been to several different plastic surgeons, but wasn't ready to make this drastic change, in part because none of them seemed to understand what the reduction meant to her. Having 34DDD breasts was so much a part of her life, her history, that she couldn't imagine changing them. And yet, she was tired of going through life being "handicapped" by her large breasts—not only physically, but also emotionally. "I think my breasts are basically beautiful," she said, "but I long to wear lower necklines, tank tops, and clothes that other women can wear. Buying clothes is difficult. My bras are big and ugly. My breasts are so heavy that sports are out of the question, and at night it's hard to sleep comfortably. People only seem to notice my breasts, but I fear a result that would make me regret the surgery."

Cindy finally got the reduction at age fifty-two—after backing out three times. Nell, twenty-three, had a breast reduction when she was eighteen, reducing her size from a 38DD to a 36C. "I was unhappy with my breasts. I really had no thought of my health in mind." Nell had wanted a reduction when she was fourteen, but the doctor warned her that she might still be developing, so she waited four more years and was delighted with the outcome. "They're the perfect 36C. That's how I feel about the matter." Nell recalled life before the reduction when she had "whales." "My friends and my sister used to call my breasts Shamu or the beached whale when I was sunburned except for my tits, because they were just large hulking white pieces of flesh. One cup from my old bra could fit over my entire face."

Although there is some scarring around Nell's areolae and underneath her breasts, she feels much sexier and liberated. "The breast reduction itself may not have made me any sexier, but my attitude about my breasts since then, being comfortable with their size and shape, has. I like being able to reveal more skin on my breasts, show more cleavage, or not." For Nell being smaller is sexier. She understands, though, that the size has little to do with her newfound comfort with her breasts.

Nell is lucky that she had no loss of sensation in her nipples or breasts, since this is a serious risk for women who undergo any kind of breast surgery. Anna, twenty, has little sensation in her breasts now, but for her the benefits of the reduction surgery far outweigh the losses. At her largest, she was an E-cup. Her reduction brought her to a 36C, and since then her breasts have grown to a 36D, which she still considers small. Anna was happy to have the reduction, because she felt as if the surgeon "was taking a part that wasn't me. My breasts had become foreign to me." She recalled the first time she looked at her breasts after the operation: "They looked excessively small, and everything was black and blue. But I realized how lovely they looked—how they were supposed to be. Now, you can barely see the scars."

Anna described the procedure as being wonderfully freeing. "I felt more assertive, aware, and confident. I felt lighter.

My head was up, my face was out. I could just walk around without being conscious of what was moving or what people were looking at. They are no longer their own entity. It's me as a package rather than this huge chest and, 'Oh look, a girl behind it.'"

As part of the breast reduction procedure, most surgeons do before and after pictures. Cindy said that she was glad to have proof of her old breasts. "I'm so happy with the way they are now, and whenever I start to doubt that, I pull out the old photos. I look at them and can barely believe that that was me." After decades of coping with big breasts, Cindy is starting anew with breasts she enjoys. These women have taken perhaps the most noticeable part of their bodies and voluntarily reduced it. The repercussions—both physical and emotional—are boundless.

Living Large

"I thought, why not complete the body image I have of myself by making my breasts the size I've always wished they were?"

—Lucia, thirty-two

If breast reduction is accepted and even respected, breast augmentation is its evil twin. Apart from the question of the risks of silicone implants, breast enlargement continues to be a contentious issue on a moral basis. The question is: can we be "modern women"—liberated, self-sufficient, independent, and intelligent—and increase our breast size? Apparently, many women are deciding that they can. The number of women having breast augmentations increased three-fold between 1992 and 1997, according to the American Society of Plastic and Reconstructive Surgeons. In 1997, 122,285 women sought the procedure, up from 32,607 in 1992. Most of the women are young and white—sixty percent were between the ages of nineteen and thirty-four, and seventy-eight percent were white.[5]

Why are so many women risking hardened breasts and loss of sensation for bigger breasts? According to plastic surgeon Dr. Loren Eskenazi, many women come to plastic surgery at a point of crisis—after a divorce, a job change, or the birth of a child. Dr. Eskenazi says that cosmetic surgery is "a modern way of marking these transitions, where they used to be marked as a collective." She believes that the increase in plastic surgery, and in particular breast augmentations, is because "our culture as a whole is moving away from community- and family-based values into a set of values based on instant gratification, on material acquisition, and on youth. Why do people care if they have the perfect body? Because there is this notion that if you look a certain way then people will love you and include you."

Looking "a certain way" of course translates to looking "normal." The problem is that there is little understanding of what constitutes "normal." "All women know is what we see in magazines or the movies," says Dr. Eskenazi. "Most women don't know what the range of normal breasts looks like. Unless you're a doctor and you've seen thousands of women with their shirts off, you don't know." Most women are willing to put up with the discomfort in order to achieve what they think is normal. Vicky, thirty-two, described just how painful the post-surgical recovery can be: "You feel nauseous. You're thinking, 'Who stuck these cinder blocks under my skin?' Your mobility is so compromised that you can't even wipe your own butt when you go to the bathroom. It's degrading. Then after the first twelve hours you get more mobility. But you still feel really lousy. You can't sit up without help. It's pretty extreme."

I met Lucia, a thirty-two-year-old stay-at-home mom, through an on-line chat area about breast augmentation. She was reluctant to speak on the phone, and meeting in person wasn't possible since she lives in another state, so we began corresponding via e-mail. Lucia was about to go through a breast augmentation, and was nervous, excited, and glad to have someone to talk to about her concerns and hopes. She had small breasts, 34AA, and she complained of feeling self-conscious, having to wear padded bras to compensate. "I have thought a lot about augmentation over the years, but I knew it was expensive and never thought I would spend that much money on cosmetic surgery."

Lucia changed her mind when, after the birth of her two children, she became more physically fit. She appreciated her new stronger, fitter body, but she was still unhappy about her small breasts. "I thought, why not complete the body image I have of myself by making my breasts the size I've always wished they were? The turning point came when I read a book called

How to Drive Your Man Even Wilder in Bed. It's a pretty racy book that a few of my girlfriends and I bought on a 'Girl's Night Out' and traded around for fun. There's a section on your 'sexual glow' and it talked about considering changing something about yourself that you don't like if it seems to inhibit you. It seemed like such a simple thought. Shortly after reading that I made the decision to pursue breast augmentation."

Still, Lucia had reservations about the saline implant procedure. "I was nervous about changing my body shape. I've always had small breasts, so I knew it was going to be different and I also felt a little like I was going to miss being small. I even felt guilty for changing my body, as if I wasn't being true to my natural self." Two weeks after the augmentation, Lucia wrote, "My first thought was 'What have I done?!' I was in so much pain and my breasts looked huge and deformed. But after just a few days, I was happy with the results and somewhat giddy. My husband also thinks they look wonderful and is excited by my new shape. I went and bought two bikinis. What a big difference it has made! I'm a small C-cup right now, and it looks very natural on me. I feel like I finally look how I always should have looked."

Lorraine, forty-nine, was in her early twenties when she

enlarged her 34A breasts to a 34B, but was uncomfortable sharing the fact that she had the procedure. "I was very secretive about it. I assumed that very few regular women do it. I wasn't a model or an actress. I was just a teacher." Lorraine had recently moved to South Carolina from the Midwest, and with the warm climate, she was exposing more of her body. "Getting implants was simple and easy. It meant that I was going to be more attractive in a bathing suit. I didn't even go much larger. The doctor tried to persuade me to get a larger implant and I said no, because I did not want people to know I'd had the operation. I thought the more normal I looked, the better. The only person I told at the time was my boyfriend. I didn't want anybody to know, I just wanted to feel better for myself. And I did. As soon as I had the implants, I had a better sense of self-esteem."

Dr. Eskenazi theorizes that "a lot of women are using their breasts to get back into their bodies. There's an increase in a kind of cyber or intellectual lifestyle that's replacing the body right now. I have no end of engineers and school marm-type women who want breast augs. They feel more like women and their sex life improves. It's not that guys are falling at their feet, they just feel better in clothes, they feel better about the way they look. And it's because their confidence has changed. But the truth is they could have that level of confidence with their A cups if they wanted."

On the Job

"I made a good living off my boobs for years."

—Scarlett, forty

Because so much of our time is spent at work, our breasts can also affect how colleagues and bosses (male and female) react to us. We don't have to be a waitress at Hooters, a stripper, or a lingerie model to experience this. Women from varied careers tell stories about the role their breasts play on the job. Cindy, a fifty-three-year-old businesswoman, had her 34DDD breasts reduced to 36C last year. For years, her breasts were as important on the job as her work skills. She recalled one boss who, when Cindy asked for something, would respond, "Yes, but only if tomorrow is a red sweater day," referring to a form-fitting sweater that showed off Cindy's breasts.

Some women feel responsible for colleagues' or employers' reactions, and take precautions by dressing in a way that will downplay their breasts. Miriam, thirty-seven and a 36DD, recalled that she dressed to hide her breasts when she entered the work world because she wanted her "work and ideas to be taken seriously. Showing my body in any way felt contradictory to that. So I went through a lot of my life as sort of a walking brain and ignored things from my neck down."

Women who work in male-dominated fields often complain that their breasts—overt signs of their femininity—get in the way, and sometimes trivialize their status as responsible and thinking co-workers, employers, or employees. After Deirdre, twenty-three and a 36C, graduated from college, she worked as an organizer for the Steel Workers Union, where she was not only one of the few women on the job, but also twenty or thirty years younger than most of the union men. "The only other woman on that job was very small-breasted, and fit in with the guys better than I did. I became so conscious of my breasts while I worked there. I felt that everyone was looking at them all the time, which they were. I would wear really baggy clothes. It changed the way I felt in my body and what my comfort level was. I really resented my breasts sometimes—not only was I an outsider because I was young and female, but I was an outsider because I had breasts that everybody was looking at. I think they really undermined my authority in a lot of ways." Now Deirdre works with textile workers in a female-dominated environment. "I dress completely different and feel so much more comfortable now—it was a radical change being around a lot of women again."

For Brenda, a former lingerie model, her breasts were an important part of her personal and her work identity. Now forty-four, she recalled the first time she did a photo shoot modeling bras. "I couldn't fill out the bra, it was a little loose. The stylist came over and stuffed the bra with some very soft plastic, like they use to cover dry cleaning. We did the shoot, and the photographs looked great. Based on those photos, I got about ten more jobs doing bras and panties. But I felt really inadequate that I had to have the bra stuffed. The illusion was all that mattered to the clients, but I felt ashamed that I couldn't fill out the bra all by myself." Brenda's sense of not "filling out the bra" by herself was a literal expression of what many other women speak of figuratively.

For women who work as strippers, breasts become a part of their identity in a rather extreme way. Bella, a twenty-three-year-old mother of one, has worked as a stripper, dominatrix, adult movie actress, and adult model. "If I didn't have my breasts looking the way they do, I'd have to get a normal job and work a little harder at it, not that I don't work hard. But they definitely saved me. I showed my breasts way before I got into this business. I was always an exhibitionist. And I did have perfect breasts before the baby." Bella no longer works in strip clubs, in part because her breasts changed after the birth of her son, and she resents the requirements to be a "Barbie-style woman—tall, skinny, with big, perky, fake breasts and long legs." She now spends her time working at private parties and taking care of her young son.

Working as a stripper put Scarlett, forty, at the center of attention because of her breasts, and she loved it. "It was more glamorous in my head than it was in reality, but it was just the most fabulous thing to have all those people looking at me. I felt so gorgeous." Scarlett started working as a stripper at seventeen, before the Barbie ideal came into vogue. "I made a good living off my boobs for years," she said. "I wasn't a good dancer or stripper. I wouldn't wear high heels, but I had great boobs. They're not particularly big, and they're not even the same size, but I have nipples that everyone loves. They're like the last joint of your pinkie and they stand straight out. My big gimmick was that I could take my clothes off and hang them from my nipples. I thought it was fantastic. I used to rouge them when I was dancing, dress them up with a little glitter and body stuff. For years my boobs were very good to me."

Vicky, thirty-two, began stripping when she moved from the West Coast to New York City and found that dancing in clubs was the only job that allowed her to make good money and still have time to pursue ballet. Vicky soon discovered that it was impossible to find work as an exotic dancer as a small-breasted woman, so she got implants, bringing her up from a 34AA to a small D-cup. "A lot of clubs are very strict about requirements for the entertainers—they don't want people who are below a certain cup size." Some clubs even hold the dancers' salaries aside until they have enough money for implants. Vicky has gotten three pairs of implants over the years, "I'm a stripper—my boobs have got to look good, and I haven't had any problems with them. If I didn't like them I'd take them out. They're like tires basically. I say, put those babies to work. It's like wearing the company store."

Vicky recognizes that she has a very different relationship to her breasts than most women. "They are my work, they are my tools, but they're also part of my body. I don't think my relationship with them is quite as intimate as a normal woman's would be because of all that. Boobs are shoptalk. It's like football players talking about their knee injuries: 'Oh you have nice boobs. Who's your surgeon?' It's just a business. They're just tools." But Vicky does love her breasts, "I love them now, partly because they are my creation. I went out, I earned the money, I selected a surgeon, I went through the time, the pain, and the risk. It's like earning a lot of money and going to buy a BMW."

As more and more women wage battles with the glass ceiling and break into traditionally male-dominated occupations, we find ourselves entering workspaces that are, in many cases, masculine. In this context, emotions and personal stories are considered feminine and undesirable. While Vicky and her co-workers have the luxury of treating boobs as shoptalk, for many of us, the less said about breasts at work, the better. While changing the work environment is a grand collective enterprise, coming to personal terms with our breasts at work is a battle with a higher chance of victory.

Other Women

"Breasts are aggressive—men feel compelled to look at them, so sometimes I feel like it's rude to other women to show too much breast."

—Charlotte, thirty-two

While we often think of how our breasts are judged by men, our relationships with other women can be central in how we look at ourselves. Dr. Eskenazi believes that most women get cosmetic breast surgery to fit in with other women, not to impress men. The more we understand this, the more we can cooperate with other women to help shape our identities. Although dialogue among women is sometimes dismissed as girl talk, there's no denying that talking openly and honestly with our women friends, sisters, and mothers, can promote a healthier attitude about our breasts.

How other women carry themselves, what image they project with their breasts, is something most of us notice. Judith, twenty-eight and a 34A, always watches how other women use their breasts. "I like to see how she involves her breasts in her appearance. It gives me insight into her character or frame of mind. I think we all go through similar stages with our breasts, so I can relate to where she is at with her 'self' when I see how she presents herself and her breasts. For example, Does she wear them hanging out, trying to get attention? Or does she hide them, uncomfortable with the attention they may bring?"

While we're quick to accuse men of judging us by our breasts, it takes some effort to realize that we as women do the same, and sometimes we are more critical. We may find ourselves evaluating other women harshly, based on the size of their breasts, or the way they show them off. There's a sense that among women it's acceptable to tease or make critical comments about each other's breasts—especially large breasts, but we need to remember that our comments can be just as hurtful as catcalls from men. Cindy, fifty-three, was a 34DDD before she got a reduction at age fifty-two. Years ago, she was giving a talk to a group of businesswomen, and as she took off her coat, she heard a loud whisper from the audience, "Dolly Parton's got nothing on her!" Cindy said that comments like this were common from women. Robin, forty-seven and a 34DD, also recalled a nasty comment from a colleague that she managed to deflect, "In my early thirties I was a bartender and hostess, and a woman who was younger than I with much smaller breasts asked me what it was like to have cleavage. She was trying to be bitchy. I said it's like having a nice smile—people like to look at it and they smile back. How other people perceive my breasts has something to do with how I perceive them. They're like part of my face, they're a feature."

Charlotte makes a case for consideration towards other women. "Breasts are aggressive—men feel compelled to look at them, so sometimes I feel like it's rude to other women to show too much breast. At the same time, I think they're beautiful and I like to look at them, too, so I can't fully stand behind that statement. But if you're a waitress or something and you're showing lots of cleavage, it's rude to your women customers. Having been a waitress, I know that you're very aware of that power."

Friendships with other women generally are a positive force in many women's stories. Carol, twenty-one, recalled a time when she and a group of friends helped a high school classmate feel more comfortable with her breasts. "I had a friend who had grown up in a small town—she was a conservative dresser and didn't like to go out to parties. So my friends and I decided that we were going to get her to come out with us.

She had big breasts and we dressed her up with plenty of cleavage and took her out dancing. She went totally wild and had a lot of fun. She ended up finding her own middle ground, but we joked with her that once we freed her breasts, the rest of her body became free."

Maya, twenty-six, and her friends started their own movement in New York City, which they call "The Strong Breast Revolution." Although they haven't yet recruited all the women of America, they've led their own rebellions, even appearing topless in public occasionally. Maya explained that she and the women she knew were tired of feeling self-conscious about their breasts. She even wrote her own manifesto in which she urges women to "gather together in solidarity. To be comfortable being with each other; to take off our shirts, our bras, and feel what it's like to sit in the grass and have the sun on them, to get a sunburn on your tits. It's a choice not to be bound, restricted, leashed anymore." While we don't have to march topless down the street with our friends in order to feel freer, we can come together to help each other tell our breast stories.

Being playful with women friends and family is an important part of accepting their bodies for many women. Julie, thirty-nine and a 34A, bowls every week with a group of women ranging in age from twenty to seventy. "Before I bowl, I rub my breasts for good luck. My friends laugh at me, but I say 'Listen, if I don't make a strike at least it feels good!' We all get a kick out of it. And some of the others even try it. Once in a while I'll make the strike, but if I miss, one of the women with bigger boobs will say, 'You want to rub mine?'" Andrea, thirty-three and a 38C, also has a special ritual with her sister. "We're a really tight family, but we're not an 'I love you' type of family—we joke around a lot. My oldest sister and I were making fun of men high-fiving, so we started high-fiving with our boobs. We'll do that now when we haven't seen each other in a while."

When you listen to mothers and daughters talk about their breasts, you'll learn more about their relationship and their identities than about their breasts. Jane, forty-four, raised her only daughter Leigh, twenty-three, as a single mom, so they lived together fairly intimately. But Jane admitted that for years she was self-conscious about her breasts, and that that attitude was upsetting to her daughter. Leigh explained, "Mom asked me to close my eyes when she dressed. It kind of irritated me that she wasn't comfortable with me seeing her breasts. It made me feel like I was supposed to be more self-conscious about my breasts." Leigh turned to her mom and asked, "Did you want me to be comfortable with my breasts? Did it ever cross your mind?" Jane considered this and said that she never hoped Leigh would feel insecure about her own body, but clearly these two women have different comfort levels. Jane says, "I remember being embarrassed when she took off her shirt facing me full on. I know Leigh and I are intimate, but it took me by surprise because it's something I wouldn't do and I still won't do, but I probably would do if I had breasts that looked like hers."

Among family, commentary about breasts can be a bit overwhelming at times. Fannie, eighty-four, is a 34B which was considered large when she got married in her early twenties. Her mother seemed to take more pride in Fannie's breasts than Fannie did. "My mother told my husband before we got married, 'Listen, one thing that I'm giving you is a woman who will give you a lot of satisfaction with her breasts.' I wanted to kill her. He didn't say a thing. I don't remember if he had seen them in the flesh by that time, but you had to be blind not to notice them, even with all my clothes on. She didn't give him much money so she gave him a woman with some breasts." Fannie joked that her mother couldn't offer a dowry, but clearly she saw her daughter's "hope chest" as being valuable.

Miriam, a thirty-seven-year-old writer from Portland, Oregon, had a particularly dramatic breast encounter with her sister. Her sister is older, and while they are the same height, the sister is very slim (a size six) while Miriam is a size fourteen. The other big difference is that while Miriam is a 36DD, her sister is barely an A-cup. "About two years ago, she was visiting me with her husband, and we were all having dinner with my husband and our parents. Somehow breasts came up and my sister just blurted out, 'Well, Miriam, you have always had the biggest, greatest tits in the world.' And I remember I just froze. First of all, I was mortifyingly embarrassed because of the company I was in. I thought it was in unbelievably bad taste to say that. I suppose I could have just laughed it off, but I didn't. It was the first time I realized that there was a part of my body she was jealous of. It had never occurred to me before that there would be anything about my body that she would want."

Unlike Miriam, some women are comfortable with being identified with their breasts. Wesley, twenty-seven and a 34DD, is otherwise quite petite. Her breasts are the only big thing about her, besides her personality, which she believes is deeply connected to her breasts. A New York City actress, Wesley often refers to her breasts in the singular—it, the breast, the uni-boob, my heart and soul, my second pair of eyes— because they seem like a single entity to her. "For a long time I was teased and called Breastley. Now Breastley is my alter-ego, just another part of my personality. It's a selling tactic to be Breastley. I've thought about a reduction, but my breast is too much a part of me, of who I am." (Wesley also noted that most of her women friends are also large-breasted which seems to be a surprisingly common phenomenon. Like Wesley, most of my friends are like me—small to medium-breasted. It's not a conscious choice, I guess women just feel more comfortable with women like themselves.)

Something as simple as what we call our breasts can be important in shaping our sense of ourselves. We're so used to hearing men use slang words for breasts—usually in a deroga-tory way or as a joke. It's interesting to look at the names that we use for ourselves and with our friends. For some women, using words like "boobs" or "tits" can be a way of reclaiming these names. Dallas, twenty-five, has a different word for different contexts and moods: "With friends I use boobs (a holdover from elementary school). In the doctor's office setting or in intimate situations it's breasts; tits are for smoky bar room references; titties for gritty girl talk." Each different name is a different identity. Molly, twenty-five, consciously chooses to use the word "tits" as a way of feeling sexier about her breasts. "It's good for me to call them tits because that word is generally reserved for those perfect tits. Since I don't always see myself that way, using the word helps me realize they really can be tits."

• • • • •

When I spoke with plastic surgeon Dr. Loren Eskenazi, she told me that "changing your breast size is the fastest way to change your relationship to men and also to women." What better way to test my sense of self than to change my breast size? Not wanting to do anything too drastic, I got a pair of Curves, a non-surgical alternative. Curves look a lot like prosthetic breasts—they slip into any normal bra to boost you a couple of cup sizes. Being greedy, I opted for extra-large. Why not go as far as I could? I ordered a second pair for a friend who decided she wanted to join me in boob-land.

When my Curves arrived, I opened the box and there staring up at me with little nipple eyes were my new pair of breasts. I slipped them into my bra and checked myself out in the mirror. The silicone pouches felt cool against my skin and I felt a new weight on my chest. I bounced across the room— they definitely moved when I walked. What was odd is that I had these things in my way, in front of me, they even appeared in my field of vision. As I reached for the phone to call my friend to let her know that the boobs had arrived, I actually bumped into my new right breast.

The test was to go out into the world and see how it felt. I balked at this because while it was fun to try on a new identity, it was unnerving to think of exposing myself to the world like this. Finally, I decided that I had to complete my experiment, so I bounced off to deliver new boobs to my friend. The Curves warmed against my breasts, and as I strode down the street, head up, chest out, I noticed men noticing my round tits. I felt sassy, sexy, bodacious; I *liked* being noticed.

Then, as I sashayed down the street, I ran into an acquaintance—a man I hadn't seen in a couple of years. Standing there popping out of my tight blouse, I felt like a deer stuck in the headlights of an oncoming car. I watched his eyes drop to my chest and I'm sure I saw a flicker of confusion. "Meema didn't look like this last time I saw her, what gives?" I didn't know him well enough to explain my experiment. We stood there chatting for a couple of minutes and I could barely meet his eye. My body language changed. Instead of standing up straight, I slouched, crossed my arms, and held my bag in front of my chest. I babbled for a while, then rushed off.

When I arrived at my friend's house, she threw open the door and looked me up and down, evaluating my new shape. "Hmmph. You look better with your regular breasts." But she went ahead and stuffed the Curves into her bra and we headed out to a nearby bar to see how people would react. My bosom buddy kept complaining that her left breast was slipping and she didn't like how they felt against her body. We got a few appreciative looks as we jiggled down the street in tandem, but we were relieved to finally sit down in the bar and keep our breasts to ourselves.

Ultimately, I realized that it's fun to play with being different—in my case, larger-breasted—to be silly, but around people I know, particularly men, it feels uncomfortable. It's a lie about who I am. With big breasts, I felt as if I was saying, "Look at my tits. Check me out," when in reality, I want male (and female) friends and acquaintances to relate to my mind. I don't want them to be focusing on my body. And when I do want a man to think about my body, I'd rather that he be attracted to the real me.

I know now that the size that I am is perfectly comfortable for me, for my personality, because I'm finally comfortable with myself. The moral of the story is not that it's bad to be a D-cup, but rather "to thine own breasts be true." Women who are happy with their cosmetic breast surgery often feel that in changing their size and shape, they are being true to their breasts—not necessarily the breasts they were born with, but the breasts they believe they *should* have been born with.

Personally, I'm more at ease keeping my breasts out of the picture. When I want to call attention to them, it's easy enough to put on a push-up bra and a low-cut blouse, but I can also hide them away. They're there, but they're not my central characteristic. Honestly, today I have the breasts and body that I want. So that's my breast story—and considering that I'm under thirty, I know that it will continue to evolve.

Women may not realize just how important our breasts are in shaping our lives and our sense of self. Just as other aspects of our personality evolve over the years, so do our breast stories. As women, our experiences in childhood and puberty set the stage for our feelings about our bodies. Once we're in our twenties, we face the struggle of figuring out who we are and what our breasts mean to us as adult women. As that identity is shaped, we then face issues around sexuality, and perhaps parenting, health, and later, aging. If we can more consciously examine our breasts' role in the various stages of our lives, we are more likely to understand—and perhaps even love—not only our breasts, but also our selves.

apples, babaloos, bags, bazongas, bazooms, Berthas, big brown eyes, blubbers, bobbers, boobies,
boobs, bosoms, boulders, brace and bits,
breastices, Bristol City, bubs, buckets, buds, buffers, bumpers, bust, cans, cantaloupes, cassabas,
cat and kitties, catheads, cha chas, charlies,
charms, chest, chestnuts, cliff, coconuts, cups,
dairi███████████████████████████████pers,
dum███ **SEXUALITY** ████obes,
gonc████████████████████████████unes,
head███████████████████████████rsey-
cities, jugs, kajoobies, knobs, knockers, lemons,
love pillows, lungs, mammae, mammary glands,
maracas, marshmallow mountains, melons, milk
bottles, milkers, mosquito bites, nice ones,
nipples, nips, orbs, pair, pancakes, peaches,
pumps, puppies with the pink noses, rack, second pair of eyes, snack trays, sweater meat, ta
tas, teats, the girls, tits, titties, tomatoes, torpedoes, twins, udders, upper frontal superstructure,
walnuts, water balloons, watermelons, whales

"The mere sight or outline of the bosom is somewhat exciting to men; and to touch this portion of the beloved woman's body increases desire. For the woman, too, this kind of caress—which must not be too rough—is full of sexual delight. Women desire their breasts to be admired and fondled, and often seek such endearments or suggest them, more or less clearly."

—Dr. Theodore Van de Velde
  Ideal Marriage: Its Physiology and Technique[1]

Breasts are sexual. This seems obvious. Large or small, breasts capture our sexual imagination. Since cameras were invented, breasts have been photographed for film, television, and advertising, because, as we all know—sex sells. There are countless magazines devoted to naked breasts. And judging by the staggering number of Internet sites dedicated to the breast as sex object, this new medium seems to exist simply to provide a means to see more breasts. Because of this obsessive attention, breasts are our most public sexual characteristic as women. But none of this says anything about how we feel about our breasts in terms of our sexuality.

In his popular 1926 book *Ideal Marriage,* gynecologist Dr. Theodore Van de Velde rather dryly staked out the breast as sexual territory. He urged husbands and wives to remember that the "sexual sensibility of the mammary glands, especially the nipples, is of peculiar intensity and importance."[2] But because our breasts are so much more to us than just sexual objects, it's hard to establish their role in lovemaking. I certainly have a hard time separating physical fact from what I think I *should* feel. I'm happy to say that my breasts' sexual sensibility is of "peculiar intensity," but I have to wonder what part of that pleasure—for me and for other women—is mental and what part is physiological.

"Breasts play a major, starring role in my sex life," says Gennifer, a forty-eight-year-old publicist from the Midwest. But not all women share her experience. In fact, the surprise is that for many women, their breasts barely have a speaking part in their sex lives. "For at least fifty percent of women, breasts are not a focus of their sexual pleasure," says Dr. June Reinisch, drawing on her experience as former director of the Kinsey Institute and coauthor of the 1990 book, *The Kinsey Institute New Report on Sex*. She adds that some women consistently experience discomfort or even pain when their breasts are touched. "Breasts may be important in terms of women's view of themselves, but what makes you feel good about yourself is different from what actually feels good."

Breasts differ from our arms, legs, hands, or ears because they are so much a part of our identity as women. But, unlike the clitoris or G-spot, they aren't expected to bring us to orgasm. This means that both men and women sometimes narrowly define breast stimulation as being "just" foreplay—something we do on the way to sex. According to the Kinsey Institute, one percent of all women are able to reach orgasm through breast or nipple stimulation alone—but they're clearly in the minority. You have to wonder about the fifty/fifty split on sexual sensations in our breasts. Could it be that breasts are such a cursory part of sex for most of us that we haven't discovered their full potential, or are we all just created differently?

Wired for Sensation

"My nipples are very sensitive and I can be aroused almost to the point of orgasm just by touching them."
—Cecilia, thirty-one

The fact is, physiologically breasts are wired for sensation. All of us have two separate sets of nerves in our breasts. The first set of sensory nerves is purely tactile, and, when stimulated, shows the signs of arousal. (That's why when you're getting a breast exam at the gynecologist's office, your nipples might get hard. It's not necessarily because your doctor has great hands, or that you're actually sexually aroused; it's a reflexive reaction.) Then there's the second set of nerves, which is connected to the deeper autonomic nervous systems. This nervous system connects various parts of the body, and can send signals to the clitoris when the nipples or breasts are touched.

During sex, we may want anything ranging from rough treatment of our nipples and breasts, to no touch at all. Heather, a twenty-eight-year-old librarian, prefers what she calls "nipple torture"—clothespins, biting—which she says produces an intensely pleasurable, almost burning sensation. Cecilia, thirty-one, requires just the opposite. "My nipples are very sensitive and I can be aroused almost to the point of orgasm just by touching them, but only very gently, almost not at all." For many of us, what turns us on varies from day to day. My preferences vary constantly. What feels pleasurable one moment can feel annoying the next. Sometimes, I hit sensory overload and can barely stand to have my breasts touched.

One enduring myth concerning sensitivity and pleasure

revolves around size. The notion that small-breasted women feel more pleasure than large-breasted women is simply a myth, says Dr. June Reinisch. (I always thought the saying "the closer to the bone, the sweeter the meat" was a crass consolation prize for flat-chested women.) "A woman who believes her breasts are beautiful," adds Dr. Reinisch, "is more likely to get pleasure from them than a woman who is embarrassed or feels that her breasts don't meet the standard." It's true, though, that we have limited numbers of neurons in our skin. So, if you have small breasts (less skin surface) your receptors are closer to each other than if you have large breasts (greater skin surface).

The possibility for pleasure in our breasts exists—the wiring is there, we just need to figure out how to make the connection. Like all aspects of sex, the same applies for breasts: different strokes for different folks. It doesn't matter whether we prefer a hard or soft touch, whatever feels good is allowed.

Close to the Heart

"Without breast stimulation, sex is purely physical with no emotional component."

—Brenda, forty-four

When it comes to pleasure, our attitudes are as important as pure physiology. Janie, a seventy-six-year-old retired court employee from Detroit, recalled the effect that an inverted nipple at age twenty-five had on her: "I was concerned about it so I went to the doctor, and he said it was nothing. I've been living with it ever since. It never bothered my husband that I didn't have a whole lot of breast, but I didn't want anybody touching me. I was shy because of this inverted nipple, so I didn't get that much pleasure from it."

So, it's not as simple as: Does it feel good to have my breasts touched? We bring years of breast baggage to the experience. How did we experience puberty? Did we feel safe from abuse and ridicule? Do we feel safe now? Do we like our breasts? Thirty-seven-year-old Miriam felt uncomfortable with her 36DD breasts for years, and still feels that her breasts are a bit of a stranger, which sometimes makes her very shy when her husband touches them. Carol, twenty-one, was able to overcome the difficulties of having heavy 38DD breasts. In fact, because she *does* feel sexual pleasure in her breasts, those sensations have more than compensated for the burden. "From the first time that I had my breasts fondled, they've been a big part of my sexuality—by myself and with boyfriends. It's a turn-on watching someone on my breast—even in my fantasies. So even though I can't find the right bra, or clothes that fit on top, and they get in my way and give me back pain, when it comes down to it, they make me feel good."

For women who are breast feeding, the status of their breasts as milk producers may make them feel less sexual. Marla, a forty-four-year-old mother of three, expressed what often happens to women who breast feed for extended periods. "My breasts used to be an erotic zone for me, but now I'm very touched out from nursing for a long time. I just don't want to be touched. I don't feel this all the time, but it's more than my husband and I would like. I get so tired of touch and I need a little bit of space just for myself. Sometimes that's pleasure by itself. Maybe not sexual pleasure, but it's nice."

Our receptivity to pleasure can also depend on meeting the right person. Wesley, a twenty-seven-year-old actress, never received any pleasure until she met her most recent boyfriend. "In the beginning of our relationship I wanted him to breast feed every night." For Carrie, twenty-four, the change came when she met her future husband. "Breasts and sex were always fraught with shame and trauma, just because I was known as the girl with the big boobs. Guys were sometimes more attracted to my boobs than to me. When I was sixteen I met my husband in Outward Bound. The first time he saw me I was wearing a big, yellow rain slicker; he couldn't see any part of my body. So, on that first day, I knew he was attracted to my personality and not to my boobs. That was a good starting point. We lived in different states, so we didn't see each other for the first year of our relationship, but we talked on the phone and wrote letters. Our relationship was based on our personalities and not what he thought of my body."

Because our breasts influence our lives in so many ways, it's not surprising that they can trigger strong emotions—both positive and negative. Some women find breast stimulation emotionally distancing. "When a man touches my breasts, I feel a little removed from the whole experience—as if he's on a date with my breasts," said Amy, a thirty-year-old magazine editor. "I like my nipples to be touched, but I hate having them sucked. There's this weird, empty, lonely feeling I get when someone sucks on them." For Tina, thirty-four, the reaction can be more intense. "My boyfriend *loves* to suck on my nipples, but sometimes I get this sense that he is focusing on them and tuning me out, and I can feel a wave of resentment, almost jealousy, when he latches onto my breasts."

For forty-four-year-old Brenda, breast and nipple stimulation is much more positive—and an essential part of lovemaking. "Breast stimulation and kissing open the door to the sexual experience. If I don't have that I can't go much further. It's the area over my heart, that helps open my heart and lets me feel physically and emotionally open to a lover. Without breast stimulation, sex is purely physical with no emotional component." Erika, twenty-six, a modern dancer with an athletic body and small breasts, agreed that breasts are "close to a source of great emotion, so it's a source of pleasure to have them touched and kissed—it's a place of warmth and love."

The link between breasts and mothering means that both men and women may treat breasts as a maternal object during lovemaking. This connection can be rewarding and comforting for some women. "I like the way lovers like to curl up to them. They might not be very sensitive, but I love that maternal aspect of them more," said twenty-year-old Anna, who had a breast reduction as a teenager. Scarlett, forty, is less sentimental about this maternal role. "I had a boyfriend who would be there for the longest time. I would feel like I had this 180-pound baby in my arms, and occasionally he'd fall asleep there. I'm sure he thought he was giving me great pleasure, but it just didn't do it for me."

Charlotte, thirty-two, remembered being involved with a man about whom she felt very ambivalent. "I woke up and he was curled up in a fetal position sucking my nipple. It was revolting; all I could think was, 'Get me out of here!'" For her, the intimacy of this gesture didn't fit with their relationship. On the other hand, Brenda, who never had a child, regrets never having experienced breast feeding: "Breast feeding a lover has always been a fantasy of mine."

The emotional component of sex is as important as the physical. We all know that satisfying sex often has little to do with the mechanics, and everything to do with our mental and emotional state. If we're experiencing a block in our pleasure, we may want to examine what kind of feelings are emerging. Ultimately, our hearts and our minds are more important to our sexual fulfillment than our breasts are.

Other Pleasures

"They make me feel powerful which to me is very sexy."

—Scarlett, forty

The message for years was that women shouldn't enjoy sex. Now we're supposed to be supersexual, multiorgasmic. We're taught that we must feel pleasure in our breasts—that the second we're turned on, our nipples should stand at attention, and the merest stroke should send us into a state of ecstasy. With this kind of pressure, it's not surprising that many women who lose sensitivity in their breasts or who don't enjoy breast stimulation feel inadequate. However, it doesn't have to be that way. Many of us, even if we don't feel sexual pleasure from breast stimulation, appreciate them as a visual stimulus, or are turned on by the idea of our breasts being sexually exciting to our partners.

Some of us incorporate breast stimulation into our lovemaking for our partner's pleasure. Others act as if it's a big turn-on even when it's not. Cassie, thirty-three, described her breasts as "props" that her lover enjoys. Thirty-year-old Birgitte struggled with her body image and weight issues for years. She loves her 38DD breasts now not because they bring her sexual pleasure, but because they make her feel attractive. "I can't wait to take my clothes off in bed because I know that men will get excited; they always want to suck on my breasts. They think that I get incredibly turned on by it, but my breasts aren't as sensitive as men expect. Honestly, I could be balancing my checkbook while they're doing it. It's really not a big deal. But I do get turned on seeing them getting very turned on."

Though Scarlett feels little physical pleasure in her breasts, she still considers them extremely important to her sex life. "They don't have much sensation. It's more of a mental thing. It's never been a big turn-on for me; it's actually somewhat boring. In my life they've been more of a power center than a sexual center. They make me feel powerful which to me is very sexy. It's what makes me feel strong and in control. I know I have something that somebody else wants."

Breasts can be something to be surrendered reluctantly—giving women something to bargain with. Janie, seventy-six, who didn't marry until she was forty-two, remembers the dating game of her early twenties. "Petting started after age eighteen, when my mother would let me go to the movies alone. Sometimes in the movie, the man's hands would stray. I was funny—I would slap his hands away. I parceled it out very scarcely, giving a little bit—just a pittance—and as a result, I didn't feel unpopular." Wesley, twenty-seven, is engaged to a man who is fascinated by her 34DD breasts. "All he wants to do is touch my breasts. 'Let me do a little Oedipus complex,' he jokes and wants to suck my breasts before he goes to work. I use them now in a playful way as a bargaining chip to get more out of him."

Whether our breasts make us feel powerful with our lovers or we enjoy watching our partner's hands or mouth on our body, this kind of pleasure is just as real as the physical tingle another woman might experience. If we don't appreciate our breasts physically, we can still incorporate them in lovemaking for both our and our lover's enjoyment.

Getting What We Want

"I'll tell them, . . . 'that's where I want you to touch me.'"
—Mona, twenty-six

Those of us who do derive pleasure from our breasts often find that lovers don't always know what will please us.

Penelope, sixty-seven, elaborated, "My breasts have always brought me physical pleasure; every inch, every centimeter, is beautiful and wonderful and erotic. But I don't like what some men do, and that is tweak at your nipple—that's horrible. I like to have them kissed, stroked, nurtured, and savored."

Having had sexual relationships with both men and women, Beth, twenty-five, is able to compare her experiences with men to the feelings she has with women. "The men I was involved with didn't seem to grasp that it doesn't take all that much touch to be a good thing and twisting them like radio dials does *not* work. They treated my breasts as something separate from my body. Women seem to know instinctively what to do with breasts. Women sense that there are times when you want your breasts to be touched and times you don't. It didn't seem to occur to the men I was with that there might be mental and cultural baggage wrapped up there."

Many of us complain that in the rush to sex, our breasts miss out. Referring to the popular teenage sex-as-baseball analogy, Nina, a twenty-eight-year-old lawyer, said that she misses the days of "second base": "Now you either kiss or have sex. It's rare that I make out as slowly as I did when I was a teenager." Mona has a simple and direct solution. "Most men I've been with have really been into playing with my breasts, but if they don't get it, I'll put their hand there. If they've just kind of grazed over them, I'll put their hand back, as often as I have to. I'll tell them, 'That's what I want, that's where I want you to touch me,' and most of them are fine with that."

Racine, a thirty-one-year-old restaurant hostess, happened to be born a man, but over the years has corrected that "mistake." Racine's breasts, which are the result of hormone treatments and saline implants, are important in lovemaking precisely because they are essential to her feminine identity. "One thing I would like to convey to men is that you should put your money where your mouth is. Most men go on about how much they love breasts, but when you get them into bed they usually don't know what the hell to do with them. They play with them for a few seconds and then they're gone. It's like, 'Hello, I'm up here, I need attention, play with me!'"

Communication is crucial to all aspects of sex. The guessing game rarely works, so ask and you shall receive. For some of us, before we ask, we need to find out what it is exactly that will please us.

Pleasuring Ourselves

"Sometimes, I have a very strong sensation in my nipples that they must be touched."

—Marie, twenty-nine

For those of us who do have erotically sensitive breasts and nipples, they can be a powerful visual and physical stimulus in our fantasies and self-pleasure. "Sometimes, I have a very strong sensation in my nipples that they *must* be touched," said twenty-nine-year-old Marie. "I usually twist and pull on my nipples during sex (if my partner isn't doing it at the moment), and also when I get off alone." For some of us, looking at and stroking our breasts and nipples, as well as fantasizing about our own or other women's breasts, can be highly arousing. Charlotte, thirty-two and a 36B, often imagines while masturbating that she has much larger or smaller breasts. "It's a turn-on to see myself with these big, round, perfect tits and all these men are lusting after me. Or sometimes I'll picture myself with small girlish breasts." Tina, thirty-four, who lives with her boyfriend, sometimes fantasizes about other women. "The idea of pressing my breasts against hers and sucking her nipples feels very sexy, but also quite tender."

Taking the time to touch and explore our breasts provides a chance to find out what kind of touch we prefer. For so long breasts were included in "down there"—a part of our bodies that we shouldn't touch (unless, of course, we are looking for a lump). It's ludicrous—here we have the potential for pleasure—why should we overlook our breasts?

Size *Doesn't* Matter

"I've never felt less desirable because I have small breasts."
—Erika, twenty-six

Many of us have a hard time remembering that pleasure comes in many shapes and sizes. At age forty-four, Brenda, an attractive former lingerie model, is less concerned about her breast size than she used to be, in part because her breasts are so pleasurable. However, occasionally she still feels insecure about having barely a B-cup. This insecurity in some small-breasted women is often based on the myth that men prefer large breasts over small.

The Kinsey Institute New Report on Sex, published in 1990, found that breasts rank as the most important element in women's beauty for half of the men surveyed. And half of those said they prefer large breasts. So, in fact, only twenty-five percent of all men say that large breasts are at the top of their list.[3] Clearly, how we think men react to breasts is filtered through how men react to *our* breasts—whatever size they are. "Men love big breasts," said thirty-year-old Birgitte, who has 38DD breasts. "They'll do crazy things for big breasts. Recently I wore this beautiful red evening gown with a lot of cleavage to the most exclusive nightclub in New York City. I had men running back and forth to the bar, getting me drinks, wanting to fly me to Paris, wanting to put me in a limousine for the night, and bringing me flowers." Birgitte had many more stories about the effect that her large breasts have had on men.

Erika had a different view: "The myth that only women with big breasts are desirable to men is just a lie. I just can't imagine why women feel that way. I've never felt less desirable because I have small breasts." Erika added that there are men who find her sexy because—not despite—of her small breasts and slim, dancer's body. But she also described certain men's attraction to her as the "Lolita fantasy." "My breasts are about the same size they were when I was fourteen or fifteen—the

Lolita age. I'm not fourteen anymore, but if the lights are off and you kind of catch me in the right mood, I can look like I'm fourteen. I think a lot of men really like that. I represent their first girlfriend, Suzy-whatever-her-name-was, who they kissed once in the boiler room at the high school but never got to go all the way with, and now they do."

Some women get cosmetic surgery to achieve the breasts they've always wanted, to restore the breasts they used to have, or to reduce their breasts to a size they feel more comfortable with. Although most women who undergo cosmetic surgery are at risk of temporary or permanent loss of nipple sensation, for some, the psychological benefits of a better body image open the door to new sensations. Nell, twenty-six, had her DD breasts reduced to a "perfect" 36C when she was a teenager, and had a huge increase in sensitivity. "My nipples are more sensitive since the breast reduction. It doesn't take much for them to get hard, which I like. Before the breast reduction I had such amorphous breasts, and really no nipple definition. There was no way I could have had much nipple sensation." Nell also recognized that her discomfort—both emotional and physical—made it difficult to feel sexy about her burdensome breasts.

Not all of women who have cosmetic surgery are as fortunate as Nell. Arlette, a fifty-eight-year-old homemaker in Oklahoma, used to take great sexual pleasure from having her breasts stimulated. But after getting silicone implants in 1981: "My nipples became very sensitive and uncomfortable to touch and my breasts were and still are numb, though the implants have been removed." Arlette's insecurity about her small breasts ended up destroying the pleasure she felt in them. "I got the implants right after my second marriage. My breasts were very saggy after five pregnancies, and I wanted to be more attractive to my new husband who was twelve years younger and not the father of my kids. He didn't agree with me about the surgery and never said I was unattractive to him in any way. But I was self-conscious about them. When I first got my implants I loved the way they looked for a long time. I could walk around naked in my house and was proud in front of my husband. But after a while, the physical problems far outweighed the cosmetic fix."

Whether our breasts are big or small, lopsided, perky, or saggy, we all have the potential for erotic pleasure. The sad result for many women who elect to change their breasts through surgery is that, while their breasts may be more visually pleasing, chances are they won't feel the same kind of physical pleasure.

Overcoming Pain

"Breasts still play an important part in our foreplay, in our sexuality."

—Lynn, fifty-nine

Unlike cosmetic surgery, mastectomies, lumpectomies, and biopsies are not voluntary, and because of their association with disease, they create a challenge for many women to feel sexual about this part of their body that they may now perceive as vulnerable. Karin, twenty-nine, a novelist in New York, had painful associations with her breasts because of her mother's death from breast cancer. After she had a benign lump removed from her breast, she was forced to confront her anger and grief about her mother's death, and as a result was able to feel pleasure in her breasts again. "For many years, when my breasts were touched, it was difficult for me to experience pleasure, in part because of the sadness that I felt. My breasts were reminders of my mother's illness. It wasn't until after the biopsy that I could begin to feel sexual in my breasts and really enjoy that. Now it's probably one of my main sources of pleasure."

Fifty-nine-year-old Lynn, a breast cancer survivor, has

been married to the same man for forty years. "When I was diagnosed with breast cancer, I had breast-conserving surgery, a lumpectomy, because it does mean a lot to us. Breasts still play an important part in our foreplay, in our sexuality. They're still a turn-on." Ann, fifty, who lost both her breasts to cancer, thought of her breasts as her "best friends." "They were the doorway to my sexuality. When I had my breasts, I could have an orgasm from having my nipples stimulated. The saddest thing when I lost them was knowing I'd never have that again. I was afraid I couldn't be aroused again. It turned out to be okay. It's similar to the way that blind people compensate with their hearing."

There's no doubt that our breasts are a vulnerable part of our bodies—emotionally, but also physically. For those of us facing a challenge like this, a willingness to examine our own feelings, along with open communication with our partners, is key in moving beyond the physical and emotional pain.

The Moment of Truth

"I was always happy to take my blouse off and show my breasts to my lovers."

—Ann, fifty

There's something about the moment that your bra comes off and a new lover sees your breasts for the first time. Mona, twenty-six, has come to expect awed reactions to her breasts, "I've gotten so used to comments from guys when the top and the bra finally come off, like 'Oh my God!' or 'They're amazing.' If someone doesn't say something to me I think, 'Okay, why aren't you giving me the feedback that every other guy has given me in the last five years?' I usually end up asking later: 'You're not really into breasts are you?'"

Since we grow up with a belief that men tend to undress us in their imaginations, it's hardly surprising that when the moment of truth is about to come, it can be as anxiety-ridden as it is pleasurable. When the Wonderbra came out in 1995, I dutifully went out to buy one (for research purposes only, of course). Finally, I had a chance to test it on a date. He and I hit it off, and later that night as we were kissing, I found myself worrying that he'd touch my breasts and detect that there was some serious padding there. I didn't want him to think that I was a "Wonderbra woman," though that night I was.

Brenda, who sometimes feels insecure about her barely B-cup breasts, joked (but only in part) about the various ways you can position yourself to make your breasts look bigger. "When I'm lying down they disappear, but if I'm over him, they seem more impressive." Fifty-year-old Ann recalled, "I was always happy to take my blouse off and show my breasts to my lovers. It was a great moment of joy. My husband has said to me that he still remembers clearly the first time I took off my blouse for him. It almost gave him a heart attack—like teenage dreams come true."

How our lovers react to that first glimpse of our breasts can set the tone for the rest of our relationship. Penelope, a sixty-seven-year-old mother of two, used her breasts as a way of gauging a potential relationship with a man. "Breasts were the first place a man would put his hands. It would let me know whether I wanted to go further or not." It's always nice to have a little verbal or physical affirmation at the moment when we reveal our breasts for the first time. The attitude we project can make a difference. If we feel confident about the unveiling, chances are, our lover will respond accordingly.

Mastoconcupiscence

"We went out on a date to the movies, and as I'm watching the movie he's watching my breasts."

—Lisha, thirty-three

At last, a useful new vocabulary word that every woman should know. Mastoconcupiscence (mas-**to**-con-**kew**-pis-cins) is defined as a strong sexual desire for breasts—and today it's assumed to be the norm. This obsession comes in many different forms, but how do we as women respond to this fascination? As with the rest of our feelings—especially sexual feelings— around our breasts, it's often hard to sort out our emotions. We may feel that as liberated women we should fight back against men's unprovoked attention even as we might feel a little twinge of pleasure. We can't escape the eroticizing of our breasts, but choosing how to react can be powerful.

Twenty-eight-year-old Nina shared a dramatic example of the mastoconcupiscence we've all experienced at one time in our lives. As part of her work as an investigator in a legal aid office, Nina used to visit prisons to conduct witness interviews. On one visit to a remote prison in Northern California, she was stopped after a metal detector beeped. After several passes, the female guard realized that it was the underwires in Nina's bra that had triggered the detector, and refused to let her through. "I said, 'Fine. I'll take off my bra.' She said, 'Honey, these men haven't been with a woman in twenty years. You can't go in there without a bra.' I was amazed. I've interviewed plenty of male prison inmates and they get aroused no matter what you do. I could have worn a jump suit and they would have still stared at my chest. There were armed guards all over and they still thought that if I showed up without a bra they wouldn't be able to contain the riot." Although Nina—who is an attractive woman with average sized breasts—was astonished and dismayed by the guard's refusal to let her into the prison braless, she complied by going to the rest room and removing the underwires from her bra with a pair of pliers. While breasts may not set off a prison riot, there's no denying that they have some mysterious power over men.

Most of us have caught men staring at our breasts, and sometimes, it's our way of finding out that a man is interested. Lisa, twenty, recalled meeting her boyfriend: "As I was talking, he was staring right at my breasts. I knew he was doing it, so I stopped the conversation, and said, 'Hey, I'm up here.' And he turned bright red, he was so embarrassed." This didn't bother Lisa in the least, who said her boyfriend, whom she described as a "breast man," still loves checking out her breasts. Thirty-three-year-old Lisha, a 38FF, is married to a man who had a hard time keeping his eyes off her breasts when they first met. "We went out on a date to the movies, and as I'm watching the movie he's watching my breasts."

Men's adoration of breasts sometimes translates to possessiveness. "I had this boyfriend who had a hard time expressing his feelings," explained Amy, a thirty-year-old magazine editor. "He used to show affection by reaching out and grabbing one of my breasts and saying, 'Honk.' It was funny at first, then annoying, and by the end of the relationship I was slapping his hand away and saying, 'Listen, could you *not* do that? It really bothers me.' At one point I remember pointing to my chest and saying, 'Okay, whose are these?' and he said, 'Ours.' He thought it was really funny, but it was a sign of how badly I needed to get away."

Bharati, twenty-two and newly married, complained, "My husband thinks he owns my breasts. We started dating when I was sixteen, and after we started going out, my breasts grew, so he acts like he owns them. Even when he's sleeping, all night his hands will be on my breasts. For Valentine's Day, I got him a cup shaped like a breast, with a little nipple shaped hole to drink out of. That was my way of saying, 'Leave mine alone!'"

Bella, twenty-three, has capitalized on men's desire to look at breasts and makes her living as a stripper. A 36C before the birth of her son, Bella now has implants to compensate for the postpartum sagging. Her feminine ideals are Jessica Rabbit and Betty Boop—both cartoon characters. "Men—no matter how high their positions are in real life—act very silly next to a nude woman. Some men say they prefer small breasts, some men prefer large breasts. But the moment they see breasts period they just forget everything. They all want to know if they're real, and I always tell the truth that they're not, and I watch their faces fall. 'Oh, gee, I thought they were real.'"

Sometimes mastoconcupiscence will make an appearance in the most unexpected places. Birgitte, thirty and a voluptuous 38DD, and Erika, twenty-six and a slim barely A-cup, shared a similar experience—even though it was years apart in two different cities. Both went to their doctor for a routine examination—Birgitte for an ear infection and Erika for a sore throat. And both doctors—men—insisted on doing breast exams, even though their patients had had full gynecological exams recently. Erika's doctor even repeated this trick when she came back two weeks later. In neither case, did these women complain. Erika recalled, "Looking back on this, it was obvious what was going on, but I didn't see it because I was really buying into the small tit thing. I didn't really understand why he wanted to examine my breasts if I had strep throat, but of course it couldn't be anything sleazy because he couldn't possibly want to cop a feel on my tiny tits. He'd only do that to a woman with big breasts."

Every woman has had to cope with unwanted stares, catcalls, and even groping from men. Miriam's large breasts were a source of unspoken conflict with her older, small-breasted sister. "One of my worst breast experiences was when my sister's husband grabbed them one day while we were 'play fighting.' I was appalled. I looked at him and said, 'You will never do that again.' I never asked if my sister saw or not, and I'm still not sure. His behavior symbolized everything that has ever made me feel weird or embarrassed or ashamed about my breasts. It represented everything about being a big-breasted woman in the world that I find nauseating. It made me feel dirty."

Ann, who lives in New York City, tried an experiment

for dealing with men's unwanted attention to her breasts. "One year I responded to men catcalling or whistling at me on the street instead of being angry. I'd say hello if they said hello, or I'd make a joke if they were staring a lot. My sister said, 'You're copping out, it's not feminist to tolerate that.' But I said, 'Oh no, I'm trying an experiment.' Truth was, everybody was disarmed immediately. Instead of having one of those street fights with somebody where you're furious, it was 'Hey bud, how're you doing?' I'd walk by and they'd walk by and we would both be smiling and that was the end of it. It was strange and probably politically inappropriate, but I had a good year that year. There was a lot less anger all around."

Evelyn, seventy-five, worked as a waitress in a hotel when she was in her early twenties. A self-described "sweater girl," she dressed in tight, colorful angora sweaters and slim skirts. "I met this older man who worked there, a very nice man. He got drunk one night and made a thrust toward my breasts with some kind of obscene remark like, 'Oh, those bambas!' I remember being so disappointed and so disgusted, and yet I wanted to look provocative." Amy, thirty and a 34C, noted that she is "flattered when men notice them as a part of *me*, but as entities that happen to have me attached to *them*—that's weird. The expressions 'breast man' and 'leg man' gross me out. What am I, a chicken?" Birgitte, also thirty, took the opposite view: "I love it when men notice my breasts. And sometimes, I am actually disappointed if they don't. It makes me feel attractive, powerful, and sexy." So much of how we respond to a man's attention depends on who is commenting, how they're commenting, and what kind of mood we are in. And even if we are flattered, ultimately most of us want to feel that we're more than our breasts.

Reclaiming Our Pleasure

"Breast stimulation response is very individual, like all other sensations in lovemaking."

—Dr. June Reinisch

The irony about our attitudes about breasts and sex is that the most normal thing we tend to feel is that we're not normal. "With sexuality, almost everybody feels abnormal about something and this is because we don't talk to each other about it, though it's all around us in our advertising and in our magazines. Everybody thinks that everybody else has breasts that do this or that. From that grows the feeling that we're inadequate in some way," says Dr. June Reinisch.

Part of reclaiming our pleasure is accomplished by reclaiming our breasts and the rest of our body. So many of us are divorced from our bodies. We *hate* this part. Another part is *ugly*, *fat*, or *disgusting* in some unforgivable way. And after this attack on ourselves, we expect to feel pleasure? The truth is, it doesn't matter what form our breasts take. Women of all ages, shapes, and sizes have the capacity for deep pleasure. A good attitude about our bodies is no guarantee of sexual sensations in our breasts, but it can't hurt.

As for our partners' feelings, while they may fantasize about or be fascinated by a woman with their notion of a "perfect" body, ultimately enthusiasm and responsiveness are the key elements in fulfilling sex. Case in point, an old boyfriend told me that my breasts were "perfect" because I got so much pleasure from them. The fact that he could make me feel good (with a couple of friendly pointers from me) made him feel better about himself—and about me. It certainly didn't hurt my ego either.

The other part of feeling sexual pleasure is asking for what we want. "Breast stimulation response is very individual, like all other sensations in lovemaking," says Dr. Reinisch. "The trick to being a great lover is finding out what makes your partner feel good. It's really very simple. It's just that hardly anybody does it." I'd expand that thought to say that being a good lover also means *telling* your partner what feels good.

But perhaps before we ask for what we want, we need to check to see if we know what turns us on. Because we make so many assumptions about our bodies, we often lose sight of what is pleasurable and we blame ourselves for something that isn't that hard to fix. Any part of the body can be sexually stimulating if the right person is doing it the right way, and breasts have the potential to heighten our pleasure. If you don't know what you like, experiment. Find out for yourself what caresses are exciting. Chances are, you'll have fun finding out.

apples, babaloos, bags, bazongas, bazooms, Berthas, big brown eyes, blubbers, bobbers, boobies, boobs, bosoms, boulders, brace and bits, breastices, Bristol City, bubs, buckets, buds, buffers, bumpers, bust, cans, cantaloupes, cassabas, cat and kitties, catheads, cha chas, charlies, charms, chest, chestnuts, cliff, coconuts, cups, dairies, diddies, dinners, doorknobs, droopers, dumplings, eyes, fried eggs, gazombas, globes,

MOTHERHOOD

love pillows, lungs, mammae, mammary glands, maracas, marshmallow mountains, melons, milk bottles, milkers, mosquito bites, nice ones, nipples, nips, orbs, pair, pancakes, peaches, pumps, puppies with the pink noses, rack, second pair of eyes, snack trays, sweater meat, ta tas, teats, the girls, tits, titties, tomatoes, torpedoes, twins, udders, upper frontal superstructure, walnuts, water balloons, watermelons, whales

"I have observed that those ladies, who . . . have undertaken the nursing of their own babes, have oft met with unhandsome reflections and bitter taunts from others of the contrary practice . . . You may imagine the need those ladies have of courage and resolution, who by nursing their own children, expose themselves to the taunts and derision of the many, who decline that office."

—H. Newcome
  The Compleat Mother[1]

Motherhood ushers in a new phase for our breasts, whether or not we breast feed. There's the revelation many women describe: "Oh, so this is what they're for!" We can't deny that despite years of dressing them up in bras and treating them as sex objects, they're meant for nourishing babies. Suddenly, how they look matters less than their ability to produce milk. And the way they change—turning into little milk factories—is so wonderfully efficient and uncomfortably . . . well, *primitive*. Every time a mother's breasts leak milk, she's brought back to this new reality.

Expectant mothers may have many questions about their breasts: Should I breast feed, and for how long? Will they still be *my* breasts? What kind of sexual feelings will I have about my breasts? How will my relationship to my partner change? Will I breast feed in public? What will my breasts look like after I stop nursing? What am I willing to put up with to nourish my children?

After eight to ten months of pregnancy and hours of labor, we hold our newborn baby for the first time. And this new arrival is hungry. Yet babies need breasts for more than just milk. Psychologist Anna Freud wrote that the breast is the center of the newborn's reality, and, therefore, key in a baby's understanding of the world.[2] Clinical psychologist, author, and mother, Dr. Tian Dayton explains, "They've been inside the mother for nine months, and they need a physical attachment afterwards and not to be treated at a distance. We went against that, recommending against breast feeding, regarding it as lower class and unscientific. Of course, we've come around; we can't do better than nature." Dr. Dayton also stresses the benefits for the mother. "Through breast feeding, we learn selfless love. I don't think it's achieved as profoundly with a bottle. Having a baby suck on your breast connects the two of you in a way that a bottle never can, because every time they squeeze or suck, it's a physical feeling. It's sensual and deeply intimate."

(La Leche League, a national organization devoted to breast feeding education and support, claims another benefit for mothers who breast feed: they have an easier time returning to their prebirth weight.)

Talk to different mothers about breast feeding, and you might think that it's either the most rewarding experience a woman could have, or the worst torture, invented by a sadistic Mother Nature. Margie, thirty-six, has a balanced view of breast feeding, describing it as "the best part of being a mother and the worst." She spoke of bonding, being a life source, and "all that love," as well as being a milk machine, drained, immobilized, and constantly responsible for taking care of herself to take care of another. (Even a glass of wine or beer is discouraged when breast feeding).

Other mothers talk about loss of sleep and libidos. And there's no doubt that there are some serious drawbacks: pain from engorged breasts, leaking breasts, sensitive, cracked, bleeding nipples, bouts of mastitis, and disapproval for breast feeding in public. On the positive side, breast feeding mothers rave about the profound connection with the human being they have brought into the world and nourished through their own bodies.

The First Sign

"I surrendered to the forces of nature and watched my breasts transform."

—Hannah, thirty-five

We've all heard the expression, "You'll *know* when you're pregnant." Although I've never been pregnant, from what so many mothers have shared, it may be true. After we've conceived, changes in our breasts are often the first sign of pregnancy, even before the first missed period or expanding belly. Several women described this transformation as being like puberty compressed into a few weeks. Progesterone, the pregnancy hormone, causes the areolae and then the breasts to swell rapidly. The breasts become heavy and tender and the nipples may tingle and feel sore. The nipples and areolae enlarge and darken significantly, to create a more visible target for the newborn. Every change prepares us for breast feeding. There's no mistake—once pregnant your breasts aren't going to be quite the same again, even if you decide not to breast feed.

For some women the increased breast size is exciting. One mother enthusiastically described them as "breasts on loan." Though many of us wouldn't consider 36A breasts large, fifty-six-year-old Harriet remembered feeling just that when she had to borrow her twelve-year-old niece's old A-cup bras. "I felt huge. It was sort of embarrassing. Just the same, I was disappointed when my breasts shrank right after my son's delivery." Gennifer, forty-eight and a mother of one, was thrilled when her 32AA breasts filled to a 34C. "I felt womanly and sexy for the first time. Unfortunately, after my son was born, I went back to a very soft 32AA. At this point I decided that implants were the answer."

After sampling life on the other side, some mothers are happy to have their former breasts back. Julie, a thirty-nine-year-old mother of two, had always been smaller than her friends and her two older sisters. "With my first pregnancy, my little boobs became a 38D. They looked disgusting and hurt so much, I could barely sleep at night. They were like footballs cut in half and stuck on my chest. My sisters laughed and we all thought it was very funny. My husband was smart; he told me that he loved me no matter what my breasts looked like. I was relieved when they returned to normal."

Even if we know that pregnancy will bring about profound changes in our bodies, the physical reality can sometimes be a shock. At first, thirty-five-year-old Hannah was upset by the changes in her breasts. "When I realized that I was *not* in control during these nine months, I surrendered to the forces of nature and watched my breasts transform. It was quite amazing." Not all pregnant women come to this understanding. Thirty-one-year-old Louise was already unhappy with her breasts. "It was the worst thing in the world. My nipples got really big and dark. My husband liked it, but I thought it was disgusting."

As our breasts and bellies grow, friends and families sometimes treat our changing bodies as a matter of public concern. Carrie, twenty-four and a first-time mother, complained that during pregnancy her large breasts attracted the wrong kind of attention. "I have a friend who works in my neighborhood cafe, and every time I went there, she and her boss would say, 'Oh my God, your tits are huge!' They never asked how I was feeling. I don't know if they were jealous—since both of them are flat-chested—but for one of the first times in my life, I got mad instead of feeling embarrassed. I had a baby inside me. That's what was important."

For some expectant mothers, the process of pregnancy may feel like a purifying of the body. Dr. Dayton elaborates:

"In a primal way, we revert to being the virgin mother. Up to this point, we had 'dirty,' sexualized breasts and suddenly they're pure. Carrying a child and giving birth is a cleansing and a return to virginity in a way that sexual abstention is not." Twenty-year-old Lisa's first pregnancy radically changed how she perceived her breasts. "I've always been a big tease," she admitted. "I liked attention and used my breasts to get what I wanted. Before I became pregnant all my tops were low-cut and tight. With the baby coming, it's not appropriate for me to show off my cleavage. My breasts are here for a good reason, they're not just sexual objects." In contrast, Carrie got in touch with their sexiness after years of shame over men's attraction to her large breasts. "I got a pleasure out of them I never felt before. It felt great to have my husband caress my breasts. Everything was *really* heightened. My belly was huge, I got lots of stretch marks, and my boobs were drooping, but I felt great."

Pregnancy prepares women for motherhood both physically and mentally, and the comfort of this transformation will vary from woman to woman. But as we watch the changes in our bodies we can't help but understand on the most visceral level that our breasts are going through a metamorphosis from sex object to a source of nurturing. How well we adapt to this new twist in our breast stories will depend, to a large extent, on how comfortable we are accepting the fact that during this phase of our lives we aren't in control anymore.

Natural but Not Easy

"Breast feeding is the ultimate experience for a woman."
—Judith, twenty-eight

Although breast feeding is natural, that doesn't mean it's easy. My mother described beginning nursing as being like "trying to learn to dance from a diagram in a book. When the music starts you don't have a clue of what to do and you've got this partner who doesn't know how to dance either." Thirty-three-year-old Lisha recalled her efforts to nurse her first child. "I was in my early twenties, and everybody told me, 'You're supposed to breast feed, it's the most natural thing.' They gave me my son and left. So I had this little person and these big breasts, and somehow I was supposed to get both of them to mesh together without anyone showing me how. So, I looked at him and he looked at me, and he said, 'Oh, you're my mother.' I said, 'Beautiful son, are you hungry?' He said, 'No,' and went to sleep. I left the hospital feeling very inadequate because I wasn't breast feeding. I tried to ask for help, but at that time, if you didn't know how, they weren't going to teach you."

In our society, we rarely raise children with our mothers or other experienced women nearby to help us along the way. We're lucky if someone comes to our rescue. Ilana, a forty-seven-year-old mother of three, remembered the woman—a stranger—who first taught her how to nurse. "I was in a room in the hospital with a mother and this was her fifth kid, but I was clueless. She showed me that I could lie down and nurse my son while sleeping, and it was magic. This experienced mother, rather than a nurse or a doctor, told me this, and that had a very big impact on me."

Because there is so little practical information about breast feeding, many mothers are surprised by the difficulties they encounter. We may picture an idyllic scene of maternal love—there we are smiling beatifically as we cradle our beautiful newborn in our arms. The reality simply isn't that perfect. One of my mother's shattered assumptions was that nursing would be soft and cuddly. "There's nothing tender about it. It feels like teeth chomping down and it's quite a shock."

Too often those who should give us encouragement discourage us. Charlene, fifty, had her son in California in 1968: "I was the only person in the hospital who was breast feeding. They told me it would be bad for my baby, and they gave him bottles when he wasn't with me. No one would help me. They said, 'Oh, he'll either do it or he won't.' It was traumatic." When Charlene developed a painful case of mastitis (an infection of the breast or nipple), the doctors scolded her and told her that she'd brought it on by nursing. She reluctantly stopped breast feeding—though it would have been perfectly healthy to nurse her son with her other breast. And sometimes we're given wrong or incomplete advice. A nurse gave my mother a sun lamp and told her to tan her breasts to desensitize the nipples. My mother burned her nipples, which left her in even more pain. "I walked around the apartment for a month wearing a bra with the cups cut out; I couldn't stand to have anything touching my nipples."

Judith, twenty-eight and a mother of two, persisted through a painful beginning, and was amply rewarded. "When my milk finally came in, it was *hell*. My breasts leaked and ached a lot. I was so engorged and my nipples cracked and bled, but I continued to nurse. Breast feeding is the ultimate experience for a woman besides birth—I loved it."

Some lucky mothers are able to nurse immediately, without any trouble. Carrie, the mother of a four-month-old daughter, was able to breast feed five minutes after she gave birth. "I worried that my large breasts would be a problem because I'd talked to many women who'd had trouble breast feeding. So I went to La Leche League meetings, read books, and watched videos. Yet, when it came to that first moment, we both just knew what to do. It was the most amazing feeling."

Even if intellectually we understand that our ability to breast feed immediately is no indication of how good we are as mothers, we still want this first moment with our newborn to be successful. While this is perfectly understandable, we might do well to remind ourselves that even though breast feeding is one of the oldest practices in the world, it must be learned anew by each and every first-time mother.

New Sensations

"Because breast feeding is so good for the baby, if it makes you feel good, what could be better?"

—Dr. June Reinisch

I have never breast fed, so I can't quite imagine what it's like. All right, so I can imagine what it's like to have someone's mouth on my breast, but I admit that's not the same thing as nursing a baby. I certainly can't picture a lover sucking on my breasts twenty minutes at a time, eight to twelve times a day, waking me in the middle of the night crying for my breasts. Suddenly, it seems a lot less exciting. In many ways, breast feeding is another setup for women. What if I can't do it or my baby doesn't want my breast? What if I don't have enough milk? What if I hate breast feeding or like it too much? Will I nurse long enough? Will I wean soon enough? *Am I a good mother? Are my breasts good enough?*

Mothers who love breast feeding have a slightly evangelical approach when they talk about it. The word "wonderful" is used a lot. One mother described the feeling of her milk letting down as "pure heaven." Another spent ten minutes detailing the different *sucks* a baby can have—that is, the rhythm with which a baby nurses. (Suck, suck, swallow. Suck, swallow, suck, swallow, and so on.) "Breast feeding is a connection that you can't possibly have with another person," added Ilana. "If it's your first baby, it's just the two of you—you just sit there and they suckle your breasts and grow. You watch their fingers fill out and you watch them get thighs where before they had chicken legs. It's because you're nursing them; it's not coming from anyplace else. It's very empowering to be able to do that."

On a physiological level, hormones during pregnancy and lactation increase sensitivity. My mother remembered that any time she touched her nipples during pregnancy she felt blissful. "It wasn't sexual; it was a deep wave of relaxation. I thought, 'Wow, breast feeding is going to be great!'" It didn't turn out to be quite as relaxing as she hoped. For some breast feeding mothers, the pregnancy hormones may act like powerful drugs. "Breast feeding is like a sedative," said Carrie. "I'd feel this wave of calm come over my body. Later, as I came down off all the pregnancy hormones, I'd just sit in my rocking chair and cry and feed her."

Sensually pleasurable feelings during breast feeding are common. Dr. June Reinisch, former director of the Kinsey Institute, explains: "Prolactin and oxytocin are hormones that are key in lactation, but are also present in orgasm and labor. Some women experience a great deal of sensuality related to lactation. Unfortunately, they often feel tremendous guilt about that and worry that something is wrong with them." One mother felt so uncomfortable with her sexual feelings during nursing that she weaned her child early. According to Dr. Reinisch, the enjoyable feelings are perfectly natural. "It's a great way to tie yourself to your baby in a very pleasurable way. Some women who do not report orgasms through sexual stimulation of their nipples, will report it as a consequence of nursing. My response is, well, you're just lucky. Because breast feeding is so good for the baby, if it makes you feel good, what could be better?"

No matter what kind of feelings a mother has experienced from breast stimulation in the past, the sensations from feeding a child are unpredictable, due, in large part, to influxes of new hormones. Whether nursing is uncomfortable or sensual, a breast-fed baby is being nourished all the same.

Looking for Guidance

"People think it's the most natural thing in the world, but it really takes work. Like now."

—Jennifer, thirty-four

For women who have little guidance and are facing difficulties in breast feeding, it's often hard to persevere. Fortunately, there are many lactation consultants, postpartum doulas, and nearby La Leche League groups to help. Both Marla and Ilana turned their love of breast feeding and mothering into careers in lactation support. Ilana described some sensations mothers may feel when they begin breast feeding. "When the baby first latches on, you can feel a shooting pain. Then the pain eases up and the milk starts to flow. Some women, especially those who are small-breasted, may feel the letdown of the milk as a painful tightening, as if somebody tied rubber bands around the breast. I get many calls from distraught women, and usually it's a positioning problem and a question of opening the mouth wider. Often babies will just chomp on the nipple and so don't get any milk at all. Women will get sore, cracked, bleeding nipples and engorged breasts, and mostly it's because they don't have an experienced woman who can help them. It's no surprise that so many women give up breast feeding. They think, 'Oh, it's just going to be natural.' Well, if it's not part of your culture to see a baby breast feed how can you possibly know how to do it?"

Marla described a problem that occurs called *nipple confusion*. "The mechanics used to get the milk out of a breast are very different from those to get milk from a bottle. The placement of the tongue is different. It moves in a *peristaltic* or wavelike motion when sucking at the breast, but like a straw when sucking from a bottle. If the baby sucks on your nipple like that, you'll know it because it hurts like hell, and the baby won't get the milk. If the baby was bottle fed first, chances are that child won't know how to nurse properly—but the mother gets upset, thinking there's something wrong with *her*."

Even after we've started breast feeding, we may face obstacles. One mother felt helpless when her daughter went on a "nursing strike" and turned away from her breasts. As her eight-month-old daughter squirmed and fretted at her breast, Jennifer recalled, "Initially, breast feeding was so difficult that I felt like a failure. Then, when she started to breast feed, I was so proud of my breasts and of us, that my breasts became my friends again." She paused, and switched her daughter to her other breast, "People think it's the most natural thing in the world, but it really takes work. Like *now*."

Both Marla and Ilana recommend staying calm about any breast feeding problems—tensing up can inhibit the flow of milk. As difficult as it may be, it's important to recognize that millions of mothers before us have faced the same problems—we're not *bad* mothers with flawed breasts if we're not successfully breast feeding moments after the birth of our child.

In or Out of Fashion

"The live-in nurse . . . didn't believe in breast feeding. She thought it was too sexy."

—Penelope, sixty-seven

Most mothers have heard the overwhelming medical evidence in favor of breast feeding. Now it's generally assumed that women will breast feed, but for years it had fallen out of fashion. My grandmother had seven children (the last two were twins) between 1939 and 1954. She began breast feeding her first child, but was ridiculed by the hospital staff. (It was considered distinctly lower class to nurse.) After a difficult start, the doctor told her point blank, "You're starving your daughter." She gave up shortly after, and bottle fed all her children. By contrast, I was born in 1969, at a time when breast feeding was becoming more popular, though still not totally accepted. My mother attended La Leche League meetings and was part of a circle of new mothers who were breast feeding. That support helped her to nurse even though she faced difficulties early on.

Still, even in the 1960s, some doctors and hospitals actively discouraged women from breast feeding. Sixty-seven-year-old Penelope gave birth to her first child in 1965, and had to fight with the nurses to nurse her baby and keep them from feeding him formula. "A few radical women who knew a little bit about it were saying it was the greatest thing. When I came home, the live-in nurse we had for that period would get angry with me and threaten to leave because she didn't believe in breast feeding. She thought it was too sexy."

Marla, a forty-four-year-old mother of three, angrily described how she persisted in spite of the lack of support she got from the hospital staff when her daughter was born. "I wanted to feed my daughter and the doctor said, 'Don't worry, you can do it later.' The nurse gave her formula before I ever got a chance to breast feed her. Today I would have taken that bottle and shoved it in the nurse's mouth. *You drink that garbage, not my daughter!* I was able to nurse her that first night and I was thrilled. The nurse said, 'Forget it, you'll never be able to nurse her again.' They just presumed that I would have sore nipples and give up. I was very lucky. I had plenty of milk and my daughter nursed vigorously and well." As a lactation consultant, Marla is now able to offer new mothers the kind of support she craved when she gave birth.

While it may seem odd that something as natural and readily available as breast feeding could go out of fashion, that has certainly been the case at several points over the years. But no matter the mores of the time, breasts always have been and always will be the best solution for a hungry, crying baby.

Dining Out

"If somebody has a problem with me nourishing my child, they should just go somewhere else."

—Carrie, twenty-four

Although we see breasts in movies, advertisements, and magazines, the mere sight of a mother feeding her child is considered by some to be taboo and even obscene. In some states, breast feeding in public is grounds for arrest. (The state of New York legalized it as recently as 1994.) This double standard angers many mothers who claim that the disapproval sometimes makes it difficult to nurse. Jennifer, thirty-four, related a familiar story, "I was sitting in a park the other day and my daughter was getting very fussy. I started to feed her and the man next to me went, *ugh*, and his wife scooted him away from me. I felt awful; it made me tense up and I couldn't nurse because my milk stopped flowing."

One afternoon, I sat in on a new mother group at a local birthing center. The mothers sat rocking and nursing their babies—there was no self-consciousness about nursing in front of others. There I met Carrie who breast fed her daughter Lola as we spoke. "Since I've had Lola, I'm not embarrassed by my body anymore. I don't flash anyone, but if somebody has a problem with me *nourishing* my child, they should just go somewhere else. I've had people suggest that I go to the rest room, but I'm not about to sit on the toilet to feed my child."

Even our families may criticize us for breast feeding in their presence. Penelope recalled an incident that happened to her in the 1960s. "Once, I was at my husband's aunt's and it was time to nurse. I lifted my sweater slightly to feed my son— you couldn't see my breast—and they all walked out of the room. I thought they were crazy." Ilana had the opposite experience. She was scolded at a large family gathering when she covered her breast and her baby's head with a scarf. "My grandmother got so upset. She said, 'You do not cover your baby's head. This is not a shame; this is a wonderful thing!' She was really a piece of work. We were sitting around the table for a holiday, and my sister-in-law—a very modest woman—was pregnant. Grandmother asked her if she was going to breast feed and she said she didn't think so. And Grandmother said, 'Well, I don't see why not. You've got a nice set of jugs there.' Everybody dropped their spoons into their soup."

Perhaps some day it will be commonplace to see a mother

breast feed her baby in public, as it is in certain countries to-day. Until then, mothers who nurse outside of the home may face criticism—something that is certainly hard to accept in a world that celebrates sexual breasts, yet considers the nurturing breast taboo.

No Easy Formula

"My poor breasts simply couldn't take it."
—Arlette, fifty-eight

Often, women who opt not to breast feed face moral judgments about their decision. The implication is that they're not good mothers if they don't nurse. Julie, thirty-nine, had two stillborn births before her first daughter was born, and was so overwhelmed by pregnancy and labor that she didn't want to put her body and her breasts through any more stress. "There was no way I was going to do this to myself. We gave our children bottles and they did very well on them. There was peer pressure, but I felt no guilt."

Some women plan to breast feed, but change their minds after a difficult beginning. Bella was nineteen when she had her baby, and stopped breast feeding after one day because it was "so painful; it was like torture. My breasts blew up from a C-cup to a double D. I didn't expect them to get that big. When I gave up, it was too late: the milk kept coming and they got really big. It was a nightmare. My nipples cracked. I would never have another baby just because of that. It took a week to get rid of the milk. By the time it was gone, I was 180 pounds with very saggy C-cups. It was very depressing. Nobody told me I was going to have so much pain and trouble."

Even with support groups, some mothers find breast feeding frustratingly impossible, and are left feeling guilty and deficient. When Lucia had her first child six years ago at age twenty-six, her inability to breast feed only seemed to confirm her negative feelings about her size 34AA breasts. "I breast fed for two weeks and was absolutely miserable. I had sore nipples and my baby wasn't getting enough milk. He cried a lot and I couldn't emotionally handle having him attached to me so much. When I was five months pregnant with my second son, I started going to La Leche meetings; I was determined to make it work. But he also cried a lot from hunger and wanted to nurse all the time, and I ran out of steam even with the support of La Leche. My milk wouldn't let down, and I became very anxious which made everything worse. I felt like a failure."

Arlette, a fifty-eight-year-old homemaker, had five children (no twins) within four years and two months, which made breast feeding impossible despite her good intentions. "My poor breasts simply couldn't take it." Fannie, eighty-four, was a first-time mother in 1940. "My doctor told me *not* to breast feed, because you cannot always have enough milk. I was only too glad when he told me that, because with the bottle I wouldn't have to get up in the middle of the night. I could say to my husband, 'It's your turn to feed him.'"

Whether a mother chooses not to breast feed because of difficulties, lack of support, or discomfort with the idea of nursing, she is capable of experiencing a powerful connection to her child. While some people believe that breast feeding is a mother's duty, others argue that if we believe we have the right to make our own decisions about our bodies, we should extend that to choices about breast feeding as well.

Giving Up Our Breasts

"When your focus used to go toward yourself and outward, it's so disorienting when this biological force brings you inward."

—Dr. Tian Dayton

When Julie decided not to breast feed, she did so partly because "I didn't want my body to belong to anybody; I did not want my children hanging on me." For mothers who are used to being capable, accomplished adults, being a "milk machine" can be quite upsetting, even if they are committed to breast feeding. Breast feeding requires a new mother to renounce her sole ownership of her breasts while she's nursing. There's no mistake here, your baby has staked her claim on your breasts, and she won't let them go without a fight.

Dr. Dayton describes nursing mothers' common conflicted feelings: "It's a profound connection with nature and reproduction, which can be quite fulfilling. On the other hand, women can feel taken over by this biological function and we may feel like Guernsey cows. 'What happened to the part of me that wanted to be a ballerina? Or a lawyer?' This is what I hear from women who have just had children. When your focus used to go toward yourself and outward, it's so disorienting when this biological force brings you inward." Carrie and her husband made this phase a little easier by jokingly calling her "the milk truck" for the first few weeks.

Sarah, a fifty-year-old mother of two, could not say enough in favor of breast feeding. "It's marvelously convenient in terms of equipment (none) and supplies (none) for the mother who has the luxury of being with her baby most of the time." Not all of us have this luxury. Many women must return to work a couple of months after giving birth. Some choose to express milk for bottle feeding. The pump required to accomplish this task can contribute to the feeling of being a cow. One working mother described the comic scenes of learning to "milk" herself, which became so routine that eventually she could do it while driving to and from work.

After years of struggling to reclaim our bodies and our breasts, it may seem like a strange notion to release that claim to someone else. While we may understand that a newborn baby needs her mother's breasts more than the mother does, it's undeniably disorienting, even if it is a temporary state.

Man Magnets vs. Baby Magnets

"You want to touch me? I've had this kid on my breast all day; what do you want to touch me for?"

—Ilana, forty-seven

Because our society has sexualized breasts to such an extreme, breast feeding requires a tremendous mental adjustment. As one new mother put it, "They're not man magnets anymore, they're baby magnets." Carrie described years of struggling with her feelings about her breasts. She had been ashamed of the attention her DD breasts attracted and wanted a breast reduction, but the one plastic surgeon she approached discouraged her from getting it. Now Carrie couldn't be more proud of her breasts and herself as she nourished her baby. "I always felt like 'big boobs equals slut.' Now I don't see them only as sexual objects. I look at my breasts and I know that I'm nourishing another living being."

The teens and young women I met were quite opinionated about breasts and breast feeding. Because breasts had been all about sex so far, it was difficult for them to accept the idea that breasts are *for* nursing. "You're sick if nursing feels good," asserted one teenager. "It shouldn't have anything to do with sex." While some worried about the physical consequences of *not* breast feeding—both for mother and baby—others were hesitant. After a bit of arguing, one holdout finally agreed that she might use a pump and give her milk to the baby in a bottle: "I just couldn't stand to have my baby's mouth on my breasts. It's too weird." Another girl worried about her future husband watching her breast feed: "I wouldn't want him to get turned on if he sees me nurse the baby."

Ironically, the physical changes in our breasts often make them seem like the sexy ideal of movies and magazines. "Lactating breasts are magic," says Ilana, who works as a postpartum consultant, and sees more breast-feeding breasts than the average person does. "It struck me during a postpartum visit with a woman who had these incredible breasts; they just stuck straight out like Hollywood breasts, except these were real! You *have* to be attracted to lactating breasts. When they're exposed, you can't look anywhere else in the room. It's because of those dark nipples and areolae, surrounded by those soft, round organs. It's as if the whole earth is right there in that breast. They nurture; they grow children. But nurturing is too soft a word. They're like the sun and the rain. They're phenomenal!" Dr. Loren Eskenazi, a San Francisco-based plastic surgeon who specializes in breast surgery, relates that many of her patients come to her hoping to achieve the same look they had while they were breast feeding. Lactating breasts may most closely resemble the firm, full, perky breasts that are considered the ideal.

Even if our partners are attracted to our *phenomenal* breasts during pregnancy and breast feeding, our sexual desires may not be in sync with theirs. Many women's libidos decrease while they nurse. Dr. Dayton elaborates, "It's very hard to have your partner's mouth on the breast when breast feeding. When it belongs to the baby, we have a sense of first things first. For me, my babies took over a major piece of my sexual energy and it was very gratifying. So, in a sense, it was a greater pleasure to nurse. The baby came first, and my husband suddenly seemed enormous and hairy compared to this absolutely pure little life."

Ilana, who draws on her own experience as a mother of three in her work as a childbirth educator and La Leche League leader, reflected that many new moms feel "touched out." "'You want to touch me? I've had this kid on my breast all day; what do you want to touch me for?' The man has to understand that this is a family and he is part of creating this family." Carrie explained it from a practical point of view. "I have plenty of milk, so, whenever I get excited—it could be sexual, or Lola could be crying—I start leaking milk like crazy. My breasts haven't been a focal point of our lovemaking since she was born, because it gets very messy. When I get milky, the last thing I want to think about is sex. Right now, they're for my daughter. They're not mine; they're not my husband's."

Because we've been trained to see breasts as sexual, it may come as a shock to watch them transformed into "milk machines." Some mothers are comfortable continuing to be sexual during the time they are breast feeding, though it certainly is a challenge to avoid a milky mess. Others prefer to turn their sexual focus elsewhere and leave their breasts to their child.

Mother's Milk

"They should sell it in gourmet stores."

—Ilana, forty-seven

For many of us (and our partners), there's often a fascination with the breast's new ability to produce milk. Mother's milk is thin, with a bluish tint, very sweet, and tastes a bit like coconut milk. While most women were shy about disclosing whether or not their husbands had tasted their milk, Ilana, took a practical approach. "If there was no milk in the house, I'd squirt some of mine into the coffee cup. It's very sweet and it's absolutely delicious. They should sell it in gourmet stores." Edy, thirty-eight, tended bar after her first child was born. Because she produced an abundance of milk, she would take breaks to use a breast pump. One night, she forgot the pump at home. Leaking milk, she ran back into the kitchen and grabbed a tray of shot glasses, into which she hand-expressed her milk. When her co-workers found out, they asked Edy if they could try a little sip. She passed around the shot glasses and all decided it was quite a treat.

Breasts seem to take on a life of their own as they go

about the work of producing milk. Mothers talk about spurting milk at the sight of their baby. Carrie remembered a visit to the doctor's office with her four-month-old daughter. "I was juggling Lola and the diaper bag, trying to put her on the table and she wanted to eat. I had already taken my breast out of my shirt and I started spraying: all over the wall, all over the exam table, all over Lola. I was like a hose. When the doctor came in, my baby had milk all over her face and was crying. I was trying to hold my breast so no more milk would leak out. My doctor had breast fed two kids herself, so she just laughed." Kathy, another new mother, woke up soaked with milk in the middle of the night—a new twist on the "milk bath."

Because breasts are so taboo and sexualized, we may feel uncomfortable about the fact that they are now producing milk, which seems so completely nonsexual. It may take a profound attitude adjustment for new mothers to view their breasts as wholesome as well as sexual, and to understand that, contrary to what we may have grown up believing, the two are not mutually exclusive.

Quitting for Two

"I cried one of the last times I was feeding him because I knew I'd miss it."

—Louise, thirty-one

It's not very heartening to find out, after all the ups and downs of breast feeding, that there's yet another difficult passage. "Weaning is like quitting smoking—except that it's not just you quitting, it's the baby too," my mother recalled. "It's horrible. It's physically and emotionally draining." Yet it means freedom from having to make our bodies constantly available. Although the American Pediatric Association recommends breast feeding for a full year, many mothers face weaning earlier—often because they must return to work. When you're ready to stop, you'll know it, many mothers have reported. One mother remembered hitting a point where "I felt like *enough!* The hard part was convincing my daughter that she'd had enough too."

Louise, thirty-one, felt a tremendous amount of conflict and guilt at weaning early to go back to work as a magazine editor. Additionally, her milk dried up quickly, which surprised her since she'd always assumed that her large breasts *must* be good milk producers. "I was upset and sad when my milk dried up, but there was also the freedom of giving him a bottle. I cried one of the last times I was feeding him because I knew I'd miss it—there's nothing else like it on earth."

Like Louise, many women recognize that breast feeding isn't just about food, it's about comfort and closeness—for both mother and child. A mother facing a crying, angry child because she is withholding her breasts, can feel torn. Ilana weaned her son when she became pregnant with her second child. "He would cry and I would tell him, 'I'm growing a baby, I can't nurse you. I can hold you, I can give you a cup, I can give you a straw,' and I would buy fancy straws, but he couldn't understand. After they've weaned, they'll often have something that still connects them to you. I can't let my youngest son fondle my breasts and he wouldn't want to, but he can put his fingers under my arm. For him, that's a special mother/child connection." Jennifer, a few months away from her planned wean date, felt mixed. "I love nursing my daughter, but I'm almost ready to have my body back. I have phases where I get very frustrated and ready to wean right then. On the other hand, I'm committed to getting her this nutrition for the first year.

I'll miss the bonding, but I will be glad to wear sexy bras again and not worry about exposing my breasts all the time."

For some lucky mothers, the transition is easier. Lynn, fifty-nine, recalled that her daughter nursed until she was almost nine months old. "Then at one point we gave her a bottle with a straw in it for her juice because she was starting to crawl and she was very active. Once she figured out that she could get liquid out of a bottle with a straw, she started to demand all her liquids that way. She didn't have the patience to sit and nurse. She made that decision for herself; she was very independent." We should all get such precocious babies.

The difficulties around weaning demonstrate just how powerful the act of breast feeding really is. Not all women have independent babies who wean themselves, so mothers need to be gentle with both their child and themselves during this emotionally charged transition.

Breast Feeding Blues

"My husband used to love my breasts; now he hardly pays attention to them."

—A mother

One of the fears we may have about breast feeding is the inevitable change in our breasts brought on by it. We worry about the sagging and stretch marks, but there are also other possible changes to contend with: lopsidedness and desensitization of our nipples. Our worries may seem superficial, but they are not surprising in a society that fears (and equates these changes with) aging. We may feel used up. Jane, a mother in her forties, described herself as a "spent cow."

We may feel guilty about being vain and selfish, but it's natural to have mixed feelings about the long-term effects of breast feeding. It's especially tough if our relationship with our partner is negatively affected. "My husband used to love my breasts; now he hardly pays attention to them," confided one mother in her mid-forties. "Of course I love my children, but sometimes I look at my breasts and feel a twinge of resentment." Some changes may be temporary. Judith, twenty-eight, was anxious after the birth of her second child. "I became *very* lopsided by my sixth week postpartum. I called my midwife, who said 'it may or may not return to normal.' I was so upset I went to see a plastic surgeon about implants. I'm glad I didn't do it."

Perhaps, like Marla, who is realistic and positive, we can learn to live with—and even appreciate—the physical changes. "My breasts are still attractive, though they wouldn't pass the pencil test. I never thought *that* would happen. In my twenties and early thirties, before I had children, they were an attractive, albeit small, part of my body. Then I had the great fortune to have three beautiful children whom I nurtured with these breasts. That might just make these the most beautiful breasts in the world."

apples, babaloos, bags, bazongas, bazooms, Berthas, big brown eyes, blubbers, bobbers, boobies, boobs, bosoms, boulders, brace and bits, breastices, Bristol City, bubs, buckets, buds, buffers, bumpers, bust, cans, cantaloupes, cassabas, cat and kitties, catheads, cha chas, charlies, charms, chest, chestnuts, cliff, coconuts, cups, dairies, diddies, dinners, doorknobs, droopers, dumplings, eyes, fried eggs, gazombas, globes, gondolas, grapefruits, ha has, Harry and Junes, headlights, hooters, ice cream scoops, jersey-cities, **HEALTH** mons, love pi glands, maraca s, milk bottles, milkers, mosquito bites, nice ones, nipples, nips, orbs, pair, pancakes, peaches, pumps, puppies with the pink noses, rack, second pair of eyes, snack trays, sweater meat, ta tas, teats, the girls, tits, titties, tomatoes, torpedoes, twins, udders, upper frontal superstructure, walnuts, water balloons, watermelons, whales

"The most frightening thing about breast problems isn't the possibility of cancer. The most frightening thing is not knowing, not understanding what's happening to one's own body. Even the most life threatening situations are less terrifying when people understand what they're facing. Knowledge is power, and most women have been denied real knowledge about their own breasts."

—Susan Love, M.D.
  Dr. Susan Love's Breast Book [1]

There's something different about a health problem in our breasts—whether it's cancerous or benign. Because our breasts are so much a part of our identity—our femininity, our childhood and puberty, our role in mothering, and our sexuality— breast complications may feel like an attack on our sense of self. And because breasts are so public and private, a woman who has detected a problem in her breasts may wonder about how it will affect not only her, but also her relationships with others.

Chances are, at some point in our lives we will face a physical variation in our breasts that may seem abnormal to us. Because of an increased awareness of breast cancer, that may be our first panic-stricken self-diagnosis. It is always a good idea to check out seeming abnormalities with your physician, however most variations are not cancerous. There are many benign conditions that may occur in our breasts over our lifetime due to the constant changes taking place in our body tissues. These include normal physiological changes, such as the minor tenderness, swelling, and lumpiness that most women experience during or before their periods; breast pain; infections and inflammations; discharge or other nipple problems; lumpiness or nodularity; and finally, dominant lumps, such as cysts and fibroadenomas. There is also an entirely different category of problems that may arise out of cosmetic surgery of the breasts—in particular from breast implants.

For years, the medical profession has been using the term "fibrocystic disease" as a catchall for many of these benign breast conditions. Dr. Susan Love, noted breast surgeon and author of *Dr. Susan Love's Breast Book,* has serious problems with this generic classification of these conditions as an all-encompassing "mythical disease," as she puts it. Instead, she favors more symptom specific diagnoses. But this, she stresses, does not take away from the fact that the symptoms we may feel are real and deserve attention.[2]

Among some doctors, the old predilection for the term

"disease" has given way to the far more appropriate "benign breast change." Dr. Miriam Stoppard, in her book *The Breast Book* classifies the changes we undergo in the course of our development as "normal development," which occurs in all women; "possible aberrations," which occur in many women; and "disease," which occurs in only a few women.[3] The concern, of course, arises when aberrations progress to disease.

Feeling breast pain—or *mastalgia*—can be deeply unsettling, but generally it isn't a sign of a serious medical problem. Most of us have experienced premenstrual tenderness in our breasts, though for some women, this can be extreme. Kristin, a twenty-nine-year-old medical student, said that her breast size ranges from 36B to 36C during her menstrual cycle. And just before her period, her breasts are "amazingly painful"—she can't lie on her stomach or bear any touch on her breasts, and she often wears two bras for added support during these days.

Even finding a lump, which is undeniably frightening, is not necessarily a sign of breast cancer. In premenopausal women, ninety-one percent of all dominant breast lumps are benign,[4] but knowing that probably won't assuage the emotions of disbelief, fear, and vulnerability. As Dr. Love suggests, knowledge is power; but, she adds, in the attempt to educate women about breast cancer, many health campaigns have made women completely terror stricken about their breasts.[5] There's a sense of women being "stalked" by breast cancer. "As an older woman, I feel as if my breasts have gone from being an erogenous zone to a danger zone," said Mary Ellen, a fifty-eight-year-old journalist. "I'm like millions of other women, you just hope it doesn't happen to you, but it could easily happen to any of us. I've watched a neighbor across the street go through cancer and chemo and radiation and it's just horrible." Dr. Love describes the conflict created for women by the medical profession. "We've turned the breast from a nice friendly part of women's bodies, into the enemy that's going to do us in. Our job as women is to find the hidden land mine. And it's totally unrealistic. What if a woman isn't able to find her lump? Or what if her breasts are too lumpy and she can't feel it? Suddenly it becomes your responsibility rather than the medical profession's responsibility."[6]

Attitudes about health care have changed over the years. We no longer tend to treat our doctors as omniscient figures. Instead, many women have come to understand that we must be responsible not only for seeking medical care, but also for educating and caring for ourselves. Unfortunately, many of us remain so frightened of our breasts, and possible medical problems that seem insurmountable, that in many ways we have remained vulnerable. Most of us do not consider ourselves experts on breast health. I certainly do not. Even though I talked to breast surgeons, cancer specialists, and cancer survivors, no one has the final word on these issues. Hopefully we can find a balance between what we're told and what we feel, and come to know what are and are not warning signs in our breasts.

Cosmetic Complications

"I'm very glad I removed the implants, and try to love my body as it is."
—Arlette, fifty-eight

One of the most contentious health issues of this decade is the question of whether or not silicone implants cause systemic diseases. While the medical community is still divided, in 1992, silicone implants were taken off the market, ten years after the first woman sued silicone implant manufacturer Dow Corning for the medical problems she experienced allegedly due to her silicone implants. Three years later—in 1995—Dow Corning filed for bankruptcy. Today, with rare exceptions, saline implants have taken the place of silicone. Still, despite the anecdotal evidence of thousands of women, there have been no conclusive findings in approximately fifteen scientific studies that silicone implants have a direct correlation to the various diseases that have been reported. Whether or not silicone implants cause systemic diseases, many women talk about feeling as if their implants are time bombs.

Saline implants have less of the feared dangers of silicone, although all implants can form a *capsular contracture*—in which the capsule of scar tissue that forms around the implant contracts and becomes hard. Massaging the breasts may reduce the chance of contracture, but it may require further treatment. Other possible complications include breast pain, loss of sensation in the breast, difficulty with breast feeding, infection, and movement or leakage of an implant.

The 1980s saw a boom in breast augmentations, when getting implants seemed like a simple personal choice. Doctors—still high on their pedestal—told women that it was "perfectly safe" and women believed it. Arlette, a fifty-eight-year-old Oklahoma homemaker and mother of five, had silicone breast implants in 1981, right after her second marriage to a younger man. "I wanted to be more attractive to him," said Arlette. Although she loved the appearance of her new breasts, she wasn't so happy that they were numb and that she lost sexual sensation in her nipples—they were also uncomfortable and she couldn't sleep on her stomach. When Arlette developed fibromyalgia—a chronic medical condition characterized by widespread body pain and fatigue—it was unclear if it was a result of the implants. She decided to have the implants removed, and during surgery the doctor discovered that they were both ruptured and had to scrape silicone off the chest wall. "Now my breasts are small and saggy again. Besides that, they have scars around and underneath the areolae and the left one is very weird looking. I feel like I've been mutilated. But I'm very glad I removed the implants, and try to love my body as it is."

Lorraine, a forty-nine-year-old social services administrator in New York City, got silicone implants when she was twenty-three. Formerly a 34A, the implants increased her to a full 34B. At the time, it seemed like a simple and harmless procedure. "I don't even remember exactly when I did it. It was completely uneventful. I was in and out in about two hours.

The doctor was a friend of my uncle and I trusted my uncle, so I didn't think twice about it. After the operation, the doctor told me everything was okay, that I should come back for two checkups, but there was no problem. And I believed him. I felt great, I looked great."

Lorraine felt far from "okay" ten years after the augmentation. "I had joint pain, flu, chills, a sense of imbalance, dry throat and eyes, muscle weakness in my arms, fatigue. But I didn't find out until 1993 that it could be the implants. For ten years, doctors kept misdiagnosing me, telling me that I must be depressed. I was on different antidepressants. No one seemed to think the fact I'd had silicone implants was important. When I had them removed, the implants were ruptured and silicone had leaked out into my body. I had had several sonograms and X rays, but no one noticed that the implants had ruptured." While Lorraine chose not to have saline implants to replace her ruptured implants, she admitted that they had been important in shaping her identity—in fact, she said that over the years they felt "real" to her. "I talked myself into it. And that was the most amazing thing. They did feel real to me, and it didn't feel like I had ever had the operation. I was so sick when I had them removed, I just wanted them out. I think

if I hadn't been sick it would've been harder to let go of them."
Lorraine described her post implant look as "flat, but not con-
cave like some women end up."

For many women, getting implants seemed to be a way
of taking control of their bodies and making what they believed was a positive and safe decision. Unfortunately, some of
these women learned a difficult lesson about that choice.
Whether or not scientific studies find that silicone implants
are indeed linked to systemic illness, the fear that so many
women with silicone implants report feeling must be terrible.
The media recently reported that Dow Corning agreed to pay
$3.2 billion to settle the claims of tens of thousands of women
who said they had become ill from their implants.[7] For the
women who continue to live with their implants or those who
have had explant operations and are left with scars or lingering
symptoms, it is hard to imagine that this money compensates
for their distress.

Caring for Ourselves

"I didn't want to find anything. So touching my breast wasn't something that was comfortable for me."

—Karin, twenty-nine

Sometimes the messages we receive about taking care of ourselves may be misleading—unintentionally or not. The information campaigns about breast cancer—particularly on breast self-examination—are one such example. Dr. Love describes how these messages have been particularly devastating for young women: "When you see a TV show, a magazine, or anything about breast cancer, it almost always features a young woman. You always see public service announcements about mammography screening or breast self-exam with a young woman's body, artfully draped. You never see an old woman. That solidifies the notion in young women that breast cancer is more common and is going to get them, when it's actually not that common, it's unlikely."[8]

It's important to note that only six percent of breast cancers occur in women under the age of forty, and American Cancer Society data show that the number of breast cancer cases in women ages twenty and thirty-nine has been essentially stable over the past ten years. However, young women who do have breast cancer are often diagnosed with more advanced cases, which may be due to a delay in diagnosis, in part because most young women are not in a regular screening program. In these women, tumors are larger and their disease is more likely to have spread to the lymph nodes.[9]

For years, we've been told that doing breast self-exams is the best way to find a lump and possibly save our lives. I know I've been hearing about it since my very first visit to the gynecologist in high school. It was gospel—of course we must do our breast self-exams. The thing is, so many of us don't; even if we're educated, health-conscious women who should "know better." Marie, a twenty-nine-year-old editor, admitted: "I don't perform monthly exams, and I feel guilty about it—like I'm courting trouble." On top of that, there's the problem that most of us are so unfamiliar with our bodies that we don't even know what a lump feels like. Thirty-nine-year-old Julie, who is thin with small 34A breasts, ran to the doctor when she found what she feared was a hard lump. He examined her and it turned out that it was just one of her ribs.

Some of us who've experienced breast cancer in our families may feel uncomfortable about examining our breasts. Twenty-nine-year-old Leslie, a designer, has a long history of breast cancer in her family; her great-grandmother, grandmother, mother, and aunts all suffered from it. "In college, I went for a regular gynecological checkup. After the doctor took my medical history, she looked really worried and asked me if I did regular breast self-exams. I hesitated, and she took out this rubber breast that had four lumps hidden inside it and told me to do a mock exam and try to find the lumps. Touching this large fake breast, after having dealt with my mother going through a mastectomy and seeing her scar and thinking about my own breasts, I actually felt sick to my stomach. I almost passed out right there in the examining room. I still get nauseous when I do breast self-exams."

Most of us touch our breasts in the shower or during sex, or we do a cursory check once in a while, but the routine of standing in front of the mirror and going over every inch of the breast just isn't something most women do with any regularity. We may feel bad about that, but there's a tremendous fear about looking for a lump. Karin, a twenty-nine-year-old novelist and health educator, expressed a feeling that echoes many women's reaction to the breast self-exam: "For years, the association for me was that you're looking for something, and I didn't want to find anything. So touching my breast wasn't something that was comfortable for me."

Surprisingly, the breast self-exam (BSE) has recently come under fire. In 1998, the American Cancer Society decided not to aggressively promote BSEs anymore because of the lack of evidence that doing self-exams improves women's mortality rates.[10] "I think pushing BSEs on women does harm by placing on them the burden of finding their lump," Dr. Susan Love told me. However, Dr. Love emphasizes, "I'm not saying never touch your breasts. I think you should get to know your whole body, not just your breasts. It's true that eighty percent of women find their own lumps, but it's usually not during a self-exam. It's in the shower, it's rolling over in bed. A lover caresses her, or she feels a pain and pokes around."[11]

Beyond the BSE is the mammogram, which we have all heard is an essential part of screening for breast cancer. A mammogram is a low dose X ray that is designed to illuminate the soft tissue of the breasts. The procedure takes between ten to fifteen seconds and involves a compression of the breasts between two plates. Chances are we've heard stories about or experienced how painful the procedure can be. In fact, mammograms are so notoriously uncomfortable, that the procedure has spawned numerous standup routines, jokes, and cartoons.

Recently, there's also been much discussion in the medical community about exactly when women should have mammograms. The general consensus is that women over forty, and especially women over fifty, should get an annual mammogram.[12] Often, younger women who are concerned about their risk for breast cancer because of family history, seek out the procedure in their twenties. Dr. Love describes how age affects mammograms: "Before menopause the breast tissue tends to be denser, because your breasts have to be ready to make milk at a moment's notice. After menopause, the breasts go into retirement and the breast tissue is replaced by fat. Cancer shows up against fat tissue, but not against dense breast tissue."[13] Dr. Love believes that younger women should "consider the question of the radiation you get from the mammogram itself. Generally, radiation risk is higher in young women, and goes down as you get older. Though mammogram radiation is low, it's not something to be taken lightly."[14] Again, you should approach your physician with questions about mammograms, no matter your age.

Scarlett, forty, decided to get a mammogram in her thirties because cancer is prevalent in her family. "I had heard this female comic talking about going to get her mammogram. And she described the two plates of glass squishing her breast down flat like a pancake and taking the picture. Then when they released her breast, she joked about how she took it, rolled it up like a sock, and stuffed it back in her bra. So I had that vision in my head when I went for it. I got my boob in the thing, and it's true, it does totally squish it down like a pancake. I don't understand how it could get that flat. It wasn't at all painful, but I couldn't stop laughing. I was laughing so hard that the technician had to come out and ask me if I was okay. She said she never had anybody react like that, but I couldn't help myself." Fannie, eighty-four, wasn't nearly as amused—in part because it was so unsettling for her to be topless in front of a total stranger. "It was an awful experience. It's so painful, but it has to be done. The first time I was upset because I couldn't accept being nude like that."

Some women feel deeply uncomfortable about medical examinations. Kelley, nineteen, admitted, "I hate those gynecological exams where they touch your breasts. I remember going to the gynecological office for the first time when I was sixteen. I went into the room and the doctor gave me a robe and told me to put it on. I didn't want to, but I put it on. And even though it was three years ago, I feel like it happened yesterday. When she opened the robe and her hands were all over me, I got really upset. I'd rather get an internal exam—where she has gloves and a speculum—than have her touch my breasts directly. I know that's what she does every day and she has to check for lumps, but it's the hands that bother me." Other women don't get the regular examinations they need because of a lack of health insurance.

So what *should* we do to take care of ourselves? As Dr. Love suggests, we owe it to ourselves to get to know our breasts. What do they look like throughout our menstrual cycle? Does their consistency change? Do we usually feel pain at a certain time of the month? Instead of poking around in our breasts for the hidden land mine, we can simply explore them. That in conjunction with regular medical checkups and mammograms after forty—while they don't guarantee immunity against breast cancer—may allow us to find any problems early on. And statistically, if cancer is caught early, the chance of survival goes way up, as do our options for less invasive surgery.

Finding a Lump

"I had to fight [the impulse not to tell anyone] and reach out to people so that they could help me, and support me."

—Karin, twenty-nine

Finding a lump in our breasts may be one of the most terrifying experiences for women, and it can happen at any age. Even though the chances are high that the lump is benign, suddenly we find ourselves in limbo—waiting to find out if it is cancerous or not. When seventy-six-year-old Lucille was in her mid-thirties, she found a lump when she rolled over in bed one morning. "I was very scared. I lay in bed for about three hours thinking, 'It's going to go away,' and of course it didn't, so I went to the doctor. They took a biopsy and everything was okay. But ever since then, that little area where they cut has been very sensitive."

Many women react to finding a lump by denying, as Lucille did, that it exists. Nia, thirty, found a lump in her breast when she was twenty-five: "At first I didn't want to do anything about it because I was scared. I just didn't want to go to the doctor and have him tell me there was something there and it would have to come out." When she finally visited her doctor and had fluid biopsied from her breast, it turned out that it was benign.

For some women, the biopsy procedure—in which the lump and some surrounding tissue is removed for diagnostic purposes—can be more difficult than finding the lump itself. Jane, a forty-four-year-old nurse, had two lumps removed from her left breast—one when she was seventeen and the other when she was forty-three. Being in the medical profession didn't prevent her from feeling afraid, nor, unfortunately, did it ensure a smooth surgical procedure, which Jane described as "traumatic," both physically and emotionally. Despite the fact that she had an all-female surgical team, she recalled feeling that they treated her concerns with "insensitivity."

For Karin, a twenty-nine-year-old novelist and health educator, the terror of finding a lump in her breast was compounded by the fact that her mother died of breast cancer when Karin was twenty. During her mother's illness there was a veil of secrecy. Karin and her sister were told that their mother's cancer had gone into remission, and were shocked to find out two weeks before their mother's death that she was, in fact, dying from breast cancer. Her feelings about her breasts were profoundly affected by this painful loss. "One of the first things I think about when someone says 'breasts' is breast cancer. And then, I think, my associations probably get more positive—I think about pleasure, I think about sex, I think about how sexy breasts can be—but probably the first thing I think about is cancer."

Karin was twenty-three when her gynecologist discovered what turned out to be a benign lump—a *fibroadenoma*—in her breast during a routine exam. "I actually felt pretty ashamed about it because I had been doing all of this women's health activism and education and talking about breast self-exams, but the fact was that I was really afraid to do my own self-exam. So apart from the absolute terror I felt when the gynecologist told me that there was a lump in my breast, I also felt this incredible shame for not having discovered it myself. I left the doctor's office, got in the car and drove, got lost, and had to pull over, and was just kind of sobbing on the side of the street. My impulse at that point was to do exactly as my mother had done, which is not tell anyone. I had to fight that and reach out to people so that they could help me, and support me."

Karin was able to reach out to friends and family to address her fears about mortality and the sadness about losing her mother. She explained that in addition to fearing cancer, she was also concerned about what the biopsy scar might be like. "I was embarrassed that something cosmetic was lingering in my subconscious. I didn't talk to anyone about that and I didn't even really acknowledge it to myself. When I first took the bandages off, I was really upset because the scar was angry looking, it was very red, with stitches, and it scared me. But as it started to heal, there was something about having gone through this experience and survived it that made me feel this bond—I kind of developed this friendship with the scar and I actually decided that it was sexy and got excited about it."

Today, it's easier than ever to diagnose a lump or abnormality. With new, less invasive biopsy procedures, this examination can sometimes take place in the physician's office. But that fact is little comfort for a woman who has just found a lump in her breast. So, just as important as seeking immediate medical attention, is reaching for support from our friends, family, and partners.

Facing Cancer

"I'm proof that breast cancer doesn't necessarily mean that you lose your breast or your life."

—Edy, thirty-eight

Breast cancer—like breasts—is both public and private. Women wear pink ribbons as a reminder of the disease, they march to demand action, public figures "come out" about having breast cancer—there's even a month dedicated to breast cancer awareness. There are also many books about the experience, including several memoirs: *The Cancer Journals* by Audre Lorde, *My Breast* by Joyce Wadler, and *First You Cry* by Betty Rollin, which was later produced as a television movie starring Mary Tyler Moore.

Because of this public attention, today there is a tremendous awareness and fear of breast cancer among women of all ages. Both its cause and the means for its cure remain undiscovered, which may make us feel powerless in the face of a disease that has claimed so many lives. According to NABCO (National Alliance of Breast Cancer Organizations), 178,700 new cases of female breast cancer will be diagnosed in 1998, and 43,500 women will die from the disease. Today, about two million breast cancer survivors are alive in America.[15]

Breast cancer is not preventable in the same way that avoiding smoking reduces your chances of getting lung cancer. Of course, there are several factors that have been linked to higher instances of the disease, including a family history of breast cancer, and the menacing statistic that women who don't have children and those who have children after age thirty, have a slightly increased lifetime risk of breast cancer. Although no cause has been definitively confirmed, ultimately, the best chance we have to fight breast cancer is to find and treat it early.

I've never found a lump in my breast and there is no history of breast cancer in my family. So far, I've been lucky. But it could happen to me and any of the women I know. I wanted to learn more about what women who are battling cancer are thinking and feeling, so I joined an Internet discussion group. Every day I read through a hundred or more messages from women venting, sharing stories of improved health, and grieving lost friends. What surprised me was that even though this was a breast cancer group, there was little talk of breasts. In the individual stories, of course, women had much to say about their breasts—in fact, most women were relieved to be able to talk about something that is so taboo among friends and family. Yet, the primary concern of these women wasn't their breasts, but life and death. I don't want to trivialize the role of breasts in this disease, but at a certain point, most women's energy turns to survival. Ann, fifty, who lost both of her breasts to cancer recalled that when she was first diagnosed, she thought, "'Oh no, not my breasts.' That quickly became, 'Oh no, not my life.'" The fact is, today breast cancer doesn't necessarily mean that a woman must choose between a mastectomy or death.

Edy and Lynn, both of whom faced a precancerous condition called *ductal carcinoma in situ,* were diagnosed without the presence of lumps. Several years ago, Edy, a thirty-eight-year-old teacher and mother of two, noticed that she was leaking fluid from one of her breasts. When she consulted her gynecologist, she was told that it was "nothing to worry about." After waiting for a year, Edy decided to get a second opinion and was told to get it checked right away.

The first surgeon Edy consulted wanted to do a radical mastectomy—surgical removal of the entire breast—immediately. Her second doctor recommended a partial mastectomy. Edy insisted on getting more information, and in the end had a lumpectomy—removal of the cancer and a small amount of surrounding breast tissue—and radiation therapy. "I'm proof that breast cancer doesn't necessarily mean that you lose your breast or your life," said Edy. "I'm a big advocate of second, third, and fourth opinions. My breast looks the same, though it's harder because it's mostly muscle now. I don't worry about it constantly. For a while I woke up thinking about my breasts and being scared, and went to sleep afraid. Now, I feel back to normal, even though the radiation tattoos are still there. I do feel protective of my breasts, and I feel sensitive if I lie on them or if my husband touches them."

For Lynn, a fifty-nine-year-old attorney, her cancer turned up as a cluster of calcification on her very first mammogram eleven years ago. After receiving the diagnosis of early stage ductal carcinoma in situ, Lynn had to decide between her options—one of which was a radical mastectomy. Like Edy, she opted for a lumpectomy and radiation. She describes the scars as looking like a "little mouse nibble" under the side of her left nipple.

Lynn's and Edy's insistence on breast-conserving surgery is an option that some women hesitate to demand because it may seem less important than fighting the cancer. But Dr. Susan

Love reassures women: "There's nothing wrong with thinking of your breasts, of being 'vain.' You've been traumatized enough already, why do you need to be traumatized some more? But there's still this attitude that it's superficial to think about the cosmetic side. When in fact, if anything, lumpectomy and radiation is as good and sometimes better than a mastectomy. A mastectomy isn't necessarily the best treatment anymore, but a lot of surgeons don't paint it that way. Older women in particular hear from their doctors, 'You're old so you don't need your breasts anymore, so we'll do a mastectomy.' A recent study from the American Society of Clinical Oncology in Los Angeles, found an alarmingly low percentage of breast conservation going on in this country, particularly among middle-aged and older women. Doctors have this notion that if you're young, particularly if you're young and single and you still have to 'find a man,' then you better have your breasts."[16]

Every woman reacts differently to the loss of one or both of her breasts to cancer. For some, this is the beginning of their breast story, for others, another phase of a long process. "I never thought much about my breasts until at age forty-two, I had my first mastectomy," said eighty-seven-year-old Helene. "A year and a half later, I had the second. I thought a great deal about my breasts after that." Mary, a fifty-year-old mother of two, had been an early developer, and had given a lot of thought to her breasts as she had struggled to accept her womanly body. "After feeling alienated from my breasts, and then making them my own, to discover that one of my breasts had started growing this tumor that could kill me gave me a terrible sense that my body had betrayed me."

For some women, a mastectomy may start a process of self-rediscovery. "Losing a breast forced me to see a different way of being female," explained Mary. "I had to reevaluate my self-image, my identity as a female, and to think about how having breasts is part of it. I had to rethink the way I dressed. I had to steel myself to look in a mirror without a bra on. I was in denial. I didn't want to think about it, I didn't want to look at it. And finally, I had to reconstruct an image of my own body and my own self that was no longer this ideal feminine physical type. It really forced me to think about myself as something other than the woman I had always been."

Of course, cancer survivors' previous feelings about their breasts affect their responses to a mastectomy. For Ann, fifty, having a double mastectomy meant losing her "best friends." She recalled: "They were so were good to me and they always gave me pleasure. My chest was bigger in proportion than the rest of me. Troublesome in that regard, but otherwise I loved them. I'll always miss them, but I know I can never have them back. I still have breasts in my dreams."

When Helene, eighty-seven, was diagnosed with cancer in the early 1950s, removing the affected breast or breasts was the only treatment offered, and there was little or no support for breast conservation. Helene recalled that she was unprepared for her first mastectomy—she had been reassured that her lump was "just a cyst." Waking up after surgery was a "numbing, overwhelming shock. Yet, there was a sense of relief that it was over and that I had survived. It was worse, of course, when I was told a year and a half later that I would lose the second breast. I can't remember it well, but it was a very hard, bad time."

Knowing the process would be difficult for her, Mary developed a ritual to help prepare herself for her surgery. "Before the surgery you're told to sterilize your breast: you're given a bar of icky yellow soap, and you have to wash very thoroughly. So in the little shower in my hospital room, I sterilized my breast and I forgave it. I felt sorry for it, I said goodbye, and I was able to mourn at that point." But even this was insufficient in the face of such a tremendous change. "When I woke up from surgery I was all bandaged. The surgeon came to change the dressing, and that's when I got the first look at it. And it was much redder than it is now. It was just an angry red scar and I was horrified. I couldn't believe it. I knew, of course, that it would be gone, but to see what it looked like was overwhelming. The first time I ever showed it to anyone besides my immediate family was when I came back to the hospital for a follow-up appointment, and I almost fainted because it was so difficult."

Ann, who lost both breasts, had different responses after each surgery. She recalled, "When I had the first mastectomy, I thought, 'Well, I'm an Amazon Warrior and I fit in with other survivors, and that's glorious.' But the second one was absolutely traumatic in an unexpected way. I thought I was so together and everything was fine, but I just couldn't believe it when I looked at my chest, and I had nothing there."

It's impossible for women who haven't experienced it to fully imagine the terror and pain of a diagnosis of breast cancer. It's clear that whatever the outcome, it forces a radical change in lifestyle and attitude. For those women who face the loss of a breast—or even both breasts—this is similar to suffering a death in your own body. And like a death of a loved one, there can be an extended process of grief and mourning which may include the natural and normal classic stages of denial, anger, bargaining, and finally acceptance. While losing a breast or breasts is not losing your life, the sense of relief at living through the disease does not minimize the real "death of a breast" that has occurred.

With or Without Breasts

"I realized then that my breasts were something I always took for granted."

—Donna, forty-nine

Today there are several different choices for women who have had a mastectomy, ranging from reconstructive surgery, to prosthetic devices, to choosing nothing at all. According to the American Cancer Society (ACS), today about a third of those women who have had a breast removed choose to have it rebuilt using their own tissue or reconstructed with an implant. Most women, says the ACS, are pleased with the results of breast reconstruction, and say that the procedure helped counter some of the negative effects that the mastectomy had on their sense of well-being and on their feelings about their femininity and sexual desirability.[17]

Most reconstructive implants are circular silicone envelopes filled with saline, silicone gel, or both. (Silicone is still available to women for reconstructive surgery, though it isn't an option for the general public.) Reconstructive surgery may also consist of the more time-consuming, expensive, and complex "flap" operation in which a flap of skin, muscle, and fat is taken from the back, abdomen, or buttocks. Currently, insurance coverage for breast reconstruction is very inconsistent. Some companies cover the initial procedure, but not the operations that are needed to refine the results. Costs can vary greatly; if there are complications, the hospital bill can be as much as $15,000 to $20,000.[18]

For Donna, a forty-nine-year-old secretary from Georgia, getting reconstructive surgery was central to her recovery. Two years ago she had her right breast removed: "I realized then that my breasts were something I always took for granted." Donna, who had been a 38D, didn't know at first how imbalanced she would be with one breast. "One day at work, I dropped a paper clip, bent over to pick it up, and fell out of my chair because I was so off balance with the one boob. I went and got a prosthesis right away. It was such a good feeling, because then I was balanced. But every time I had to put on or take off the prosthesis, I thought *cancer.* A week after I got it, I made the plastic surgeon appointment and went in to see about reconstruction."

Donna decided she "wanted cleavage for Christmas," and had reconstructive surgery on December 22nd. On Christmas morning, "the first thing I did when I woke up was take my nightgown off, push my arms together, and look down to see I had cleavage. That was so important for me in my healing process. I know it's not the same as the original boob. But to me, I look down now, and scars and all, it's beautiful. I have cleavage. My other one is uplifted, it's the breast of an eighteen year old."

Though reconstructive surgery with an implant may be done on an outpatient basis, it is not always as simple as it sounds. Possible complications mean that many women choose prosthetics over surgery. Prosthetic devices may be made from foam or other materials, but most often they are skin-colored, silicone structures shaped like breasts that can be tucked into bras. Helene, eighty-seven, recalled that "wearing the prostheses was a partial solution, but hardly a very satisfactory one.

When I asked the surgeon who had done the mastectomies whether there was any procedure for substituting for breasts, he laughed, and said, 'You're forty-two, you have a husband, you have two children, why in the world would you be worried about breasts?' He made me feel like a fool. I never asked again."

As a large-breasted woman, Mary learned that she would require an implant and a reduction, which would be an extensive, not to mention painful, surgical procedure, likely leaving her with little sensation in the remaining breast. Although Mary said she wanted to be "a whole physical woman again," she decided not to undergo further surgery. Instead, she uses a prosthetic breast, which she wears inside her bras. "It's a pain to have to maneuver this thing all the time. It has to go in and out of every bra. It has to be there in the morning ready for me. And yet it does seem like part of me. Sometimes, I used to even forget which was the real breast and which was the fake breast. I'm conflicted about it—I feel that it's my friend and my enemy because it helps me put forward that conforming female image, which, for my life the way it is now, I need. But I know that it's fraudulent."

Some women end up choosing to go without implants or a prosthesis. Gloria, fifty-five, opted to get an implant after her mastectomy, but it "didn't take." The implant encapsulated and became hard and painful, so she had it removed and never went back for a second operation. Now working as a volunteer at the New York City-based organization SHARE: Self-Help for Women with Breast or Ovarian Cancer, Gloria has come to terms with her new body. Though she has a prosthesis, she always hated wearing a bra, so in general she goes braless and leaves the prosthesis at home. The difference is noticeable, but Gloria doesn't mind being public about her mastectomy.

Deciding whether or not to compensate for a lost breast is an individual decision for each woman. Some believe that it is important to go without a prosthetic breast, to be present as a breast cancer survivor. Others, like Donna, feel that wearing a prosthetic breast or getting reconstructive surgery is important in surviving cancer. Because of the public and private nature of breasts, a deeply personal decision like this becomes public and political. Should breast cancer survivors identify themselves as such by going without a prosthetic breast or reconstructive surgery, or should they move beyond it? While nothing will ever emotionally or physically compensate for a lost breast, each woman must decide for herself. There are no easy answers.

Redefining Our Sexuality

"I would say that after I had the reconstruction, our sex life improved."

—Donna, forty-nine

Many women feel frustrated by the lack of honest discussion about the impact of mastectomies on their sex lives. How a woman's partner reacts is, of course, important in the healing process. Helene, eighty-seven, recalled, "My husband, by way of being supportive, emphasized that it was not important to him at all. But it became obvious that it *was* very important. It had an immediate effect on our sexual relationship, one that was never really completely reversed. He died about seven years after the mastectomies. Years later, when I had another relationship, the absence of breasts was again a severe deficiency in our lovemaking, although again, he denied that it meant anything significant to him. It wasn't true." Whether or not Helene's partners' desires were negatively affected by her double mastectomy, her own grief made it difficult for her to trust their expressions of sexual interest.

For many women it's hard to feel pleasure in an area that

has been under attack. Physically, the severing of the nerves in the breast can leave the scar feeling numb and prickly— somewhat like the feeling you get when your foot falls asleep. Mary said of her scar, "It does not feel sexy. It feels destroyed. It feels like my body has been desecrated. It makes me more protective of the breast I have left." Donna, who chose to get reconstructive surgery, felt a significant increase in pleasure after the surgery. "I didn't realize how much my breasts were a part of my sexuality. I took it for granted. I would say that after I had the reconstruction, our sex life improved."

For Ann and her husband, her breasts were central in their lovemaking and their day-to-day life. "I used to play 'top-less waitress' with my husband when I brought dinner to him. I would just wear a T-shirt and black underwear, and would lift up the shirt while delivering the food. It was sad when I couldn't do that anymore." Although Ann said that her husband has been supportive throughout her illness and recovery, he still hasn't seen her chest. "In the beginning, when I had the first mastectomy, he was very uncomfortable with the scar and didn't want to look. When I had the second mastectomy, I was very uncomfortable with how it looked without breasts there. So the whole thing became impossible. To this day, I haven't shown him my chest. Plus, it gets harder after time. I think neither of us really knows how to propose it, so I usually wear some sort of T-shirt when I go to bed. I'm not sure that I even want to try to show him."

Gloria, fifty-five, still feels sexual despite her mastectomy. A single New Yorker, she hasn't let her surgery stop her from dating. "The men I've dated in the past fifteen years have been great about dealing with this. I'm much more protective of myself and more selective—I don't want to find myself with someone who rejects me because he can't handle this. I size up the man and tell him before things get hot and heavy. So far, they've reacted by saying that it didn't make a difference—and I don't think that was just a line. Now, I've just met someone new and after four dates I know the chemistry is great. His mom died of breast cancer, so it was hard to tell him, but he took it very well."

A mastectomy, or even a lumpectomy, can create a tremendous challenge for women to be able to see themselves as sexy in a society that so values young, healthy bodies. There's also the physical reality that it may be painful or uncomfortable to be touched near the mastectomy or lumpectomy scar. While the support of a partner can be a powerful healer, some women can't count on that person to understand and cope with the changes. Other women who are single find that a mastectomy doesn't necessarily mean the end of their sexual life. Dealing with sexuality in the face of breast cancer forces women to address the question of how they can be sexual and sexually desirable, with or without their breasts.

Survivors

"Over the years I have adjusted to the fact that when I'm fully clothed there isn't much difference between the way I look and the way other women look."
—Helene, eighty-seven

Although, as Harriet, a fifty-six-year-old breast cancer "survivor" said, "You don't know until you die of something else that you 'survived' breast cancer," survival rates continue to improve. But even as more and more women are living through the disease, the long-term effects on their lives are profound. For Helene, eighty-seven, the pain is still present. "I still feel as if I'm mutilated, and I don't expose myself when I'm in a dressing room at a swimming pool or anywhere else because I feel that the scars are ugly. I don't like imposing them on other people. I think that over the years I have adjusted to the fact that when I'm fully clothed there isn't much difference between the way I look and the way other women look. I avoid useless regrets and self-pity, but if I allow myself to think of what the cost of losing my breasts has been in terms of my relationships with the men I loved, I would give a great deal to have it to do again. It made a very significant difference in my relationships, and it was a loss for them as well as for me. I'd certainly love to have a chance to do it again with both breasts intact."

After going through the crisis of fighting cancer, many women find that it is something they simply have to learn to live with—with varying degrees of comfort. Lynn, who had a lumpectomy, explained, "When I think about my breasts now, I tend to see them as loaded guns and wonder, 'Is the other one going to go off?' I'm a little afraid. I don't know quite what to expect of them. They're so sensitive and so vulnerable. And I'm very protective of them." Harriet, on the other hand, has managed to define herself outside of the cancer, even though she had a double mastectomy. "It's always there. It's always in the background somewhere. But it's been five years and I'm fine. I don't think of it every minute of the day anymore."

All breast cancer survivors are forced to develop different ways of looking at their bodies. For Donna, getting reconstructive surgery has allowed her to be more open with friends and family about her experience with cancer. "I went to visit my daughter right after my reconstructive surgery, and when her girlfriends came over, she'd say, 'Come on, look at my mom's new boob. Someday we may have to face this.' I felt good that I could show them—the boob is back, and it's fine. And if, God forbid, this ever happens to you, it's not the end of the world." Ann, who decided not to get reconstructive surgery or wear prostheses, found her own way to mark her survival. "On the right side of my chest, I put a tattoo of a nipple and a gold ring. Each year, I add a gold ring—a ring for the year I found the cancer, and then for all the years I survived. And I'm hoping those rings will go down my chest, down my leg, up my leg, and around."

Mary's recovery after the loss of her left breast included writing an unpublished memoir about her relationship to her breasts. She recalled wishing as a teenager that a fairy would wave a magic wand and make her D-cup breasts a more manageable size. "If at this point, a fairy came along and said, 'I'm going to wave a magic wand and you're going to have two beautiful C breasts,' I would have to think about it. I don't know whether I would jump for it right away, because I've gone through this whole process of rethinking my body image, rethinking who I am, and it would mean doing all that work over again to all of a sudden be a normal female physical person."

I am moved by these survivors' optimism, honesty, and strength—all essential ingredients for survival. Sadly, so many of us have an adversarial relationship with our bodies—our breasts included. Because breast diseases, especially cancer, are so mysterious, many of us have come to fear our breasts. After all, it seems that the primary risk factor for breast cancer is simply being a woman. Dr. Love encourages women to "take back" their breasts. "Women need to really question the information they're getting about their breasts and their bodies. One of my big soapboxes right now is that medicine is a work in progress. We're only ever working on our best guess at the moment. Stay tuned because it will probably change. The public doesn't always realize that. We have to be very careful about not just accepting information that we get from physicians or the media at face value, but really questioning it."[19]

We live in a society that sends us extremely confusing

messages. On the one hand, we're surrounded with more breasts than we know what to do with. On the other, breasts are rarely partnered with honest dialogue. As Harriet, a fifty-six-year-old breast cancer survivor said of our interview, "This is a chance to talk about something that no one wants to talk about with me. Not a single one of my friends has asked me what I look like now. No one but my husband has seen my chest. Ever. And that feels very isolating. Women don't generally show each other their chests; that's a forbidden thing. I had never seen an ordinary breast until I got breast cancer and people showed me what their reconstruction was like." If, instead of allowing breasts to be a taboo subject, we talk about our breasts—not just in relation to health issues, but in all areas of our lives—chances are, we will develop healthier attitudes. While that is no guarantee of healthy breasts, we would be more likely to take better care of ourselves, and better equipped to respect our bodies as they are.

apples, babaloos, bags, bazongas, bazooms, Berthas, big brown eyes, blubbers, bobbers, boobies, boobs, bosoms, boulders, brace and bits, breastices, Bristol City, bubs, buckets, buds, buffers, bumpers, bust, cans, cantaloupes, cassabas, cat and kitties, catheads, cha chas, charlies, charms, chest, chestnuts, cliff, coconuts, cups, dairies, diddies, dinners, doorknobs, droopers, dumplings, eyes, fried eggs, gazombas, globes, gondolas, grapefruits, ha has, Harry and Junes, headlights, hooters, ice cream scoops, jerseycities, jugs, kajoobies, knobs, knockers, lemons, love pillows, lungs, mammae, mammary glands, maracas 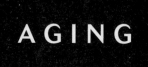 ons, milk bottles, ce ones, nipples, peaches, pumps, puppies with the pink noses, rack, second pair of eyes, snack trays, sweater meat, ta tas, teats, the girls, tits, titties, tomatoes, torpedoes, twins, udders, upper frontal superstructure, walnuts, water balloons, watermelons, whales

"I have everything I had twenty years ago, only it's a little bit lower."

—Gypsy Rose Lee (striptease artist)
 Quoted in *Wild Words from Wild Women* [1]

We live in a society that fears aging. Older women are often treated as if they are "disposable"—after all, the logic goes, when we've aged, we're no longer viable sex partners or child-bearers. Both men and women propagate the destructive attitude that the first wrinkle or gray hair is the beginning of the end. In her book *The Fountain of Age*, Betty Friedan explodes some of the prejudices about aging in the same way that she reexamined the myth of the mindlessly happy house-wife in *The Feminine Mystique*. Friedan writes that the "Third Age" (post-career and kids) may be the age of true creativity—even of evolution. She believes that we can continue to lead rewarding lives and also grow intellectually and emotionally. [2]

Sadly, as women we have few positive models for aging—we move into despair, not wisdom. The ideal is to look so young that we start to feel as if we're aging in our mid-twenties. And in terms of our breasts, that's particularly true. Despite the predominance of talk about size, I found that most women were more concerned with the appearance of stretch marks and sagging. I heard women from their twenties through their eighties express fears about the changes in their breasts. At age twenty-eight, it might seem easy for me to talk about how we should accept our aging bodies, but I know that I need to remind myself of my own advice.

When I called seventy-six-year-old Janie, she was shocked that her niece recommended that I talk to her about her breasts. Not because she was scandalized by the idea of a book about breasts, but because, as she put it, "Would I fit with this? I'm so old!" I explained that I was interested in hearing from women and girls of all ages, and after she reminded me several more times that she was "old, old, old!" she started talking. A retired court worker, Janie told me about the days of stuffing her bra to go out dancing at the Graystone Ballroom in Detroit where Duke Ellington and Count Basie performed. She shared stories about dating young men with hands that strayed; her fear of an inverted nipple at age twenty-five; and in her forties, marrying a man who playfully described her B-cup breasts as "fried eggs." Janie "fit in" perfectly. But her surprise at being interviewed is indicative of the notion that older women aren't part of the family of women.

In later years, as during puberty, our breasts change in response to hormonal fluctuations. For some women, menopause can bring an increase in breast size. Harriet, a fifty-six-year-old medical secretary, was a 34AA until her late forties. "My breasts were so small that I never thought of them as *real* breasts. They never had a breast shape until they fattened up a bit and started to sag. For me, aging was almost like developing." According to health care educator Dr. Miriam Stoppard, author of *The Breast Book*, a possible explanation for this kind of growth is the increasing number of menstrual cycles in which we don't ovulate. During these cycles there's no progesterone to control the effect of estrogen. The breasts are therefore exposed to prolonged periods of unopposed estrogen stimulation, which causes additional swelling of the remaining glands in the breast and an increase in fat cells. As a result, breasts may be tender and even painful at menopause.[3]

Most of us, however, don't anticipate breast growth in our later years. We are more likely to fear the opposite—the dreaded sag. In older women, a drop in the level of estrogen causes breasts to droop and flatten—the larger the breasts the more they sag. This is because the connective tissue in the breast is composed of a fibrous protein called collagen which gets dehydrated and inelastic without estrogen. Once the collagen has lost its shape, it will never return to its former state.

Beyond this scientific explanation, we have a concrete way of measuring the aging of our breasts: the masochistic pencil test. Molly, twenty-five, explained, "An acquaintance of mine with really big boobs told me that she gave herself the pencil test and that she had passed. And I, not knowing, said, 'What's the pencil test?' And she said, 'Well, it's to see if your breasts are too saggy or not.' Passing means that the pencil, when put under your breast, falls out, drops to the ground. I went home, got a pencil, and I gave myself the pencil test, and it stayed there in a vice-like grip. So I failed the pencil test. It means that I have imperfect breasts. My breasts fail. So, there you have it." Andrea, a thirty-three-year-old photographer with 38C breasts, has also done the infamous test: "The pencil test, forget about it! My sisters and I jokingly did that. I mean I could fit a pencil *case*. They really do hang. But I don't necessarily think there's anything wrong with that."

The first pangs of aging hit some women when they see their daughters coming of age. Jane, a forty-four-year-old nurse, recalled that when she watched her daughter Leigh, now twenty-three, go through puberty, she was in "mourning" for

228

her former breasts. "I remember she stayed with her father for the summer, which she always did. And when she came back, I passed her in the airport and didn't recognize her. She had full breasts. She looked like a woman. It seemed to me that it happened so quickly. It's funny, I stopped getting whistled at . . ." Leigh jumped in to add, "around the same time that I started getting it." Jane laughed in agreement and continued, "You were constant whistle material. It was funny walking with you, I'd hear a whistle and I wasn't sure who it was for. But for the past five years or so, there's been no question. And that's kind of funny, but I'm real proud of you." She paused, "I *think* I'm comfortable with it."

Several years ago Jane dated a man who offered to pay for surgery to lift her breasts. "When I saw a plastic surgeon about having my breasts fixed, he looked at them and shook his head. All I wanted was an augmentation, hoping that that would just lift them up. He said I'd have to have a rather complex breast lift—a *mastopexy*—with cutting around the nipples, quite extensive. I was pretty embarrassed. It's sad and I feel a bit like my body is betraying me. I never thought I would age like this. Being forty-four is fine, but I really wish my skin and breasts were not so aged."

Women of all ages critically inspect their bodies for signs of aging, and many are frustrated by the changes they see. "I'm young, but my breasts have always been saggy," says Molly. "Ever since they grew they've been shaped like this, but I still feel like it makes me seem old. When I hear older women talking about how their breasts are starting to sag, I have no sympathy because mine have always been like this. I never knew those young, teenage days of the firm breast." Marie, a twenty-nine-year-old editor, confided, "After losing weight, I went from a C to a B. Now that I'm smaller and older, I'm starting to sag a little, so my bra seems like a necessity." She paused for a moment to consider what she'd just said, "How do you like the way I conflated myself and my breasts? *I'm* not starting to sag, my *tits* are!" Eighty-four-year-old Fannie, a retired teacher who now works as a mediator, is sometimes impatient with her changing body. "I'm very short. I was always five feet tall, but now I'm shrinking. So what's happening is that my bust and my waist are coming together and it's so frustrating. Especially when I want my breasts to be up high and they're headed down. It's hard for me to button my trousers because the bust comes down. I have to watch out! Lately, I've been taking estrogen to treat osteoporosis so my breasts got fuller again. I'm happy, because now they feel more like they used to."

Then there are women who experience almost no difference in their older breasts. "Strangely enough, I've never seen a change in my breasts," said sixty-seven-year-old Penelope, a mother of two and a 34B. "They look the same to me. And I've always had a certain pride about my breasts. When I was in the hospital nursing my children and people saw my breasts they all said I had great color and amazing nipples. They were very erect and quite big. It was just something people admired and something I was always proud of. I haven't noticed my breasts sagging and aging. I happen to think they're quite beautiful." And seventy-six-year-old Lucille, a mother of one and also a 34B who plays tennis, dances, and does yoga, said proudly, "My boobs aren't hanging down to my stomach. They're not perky, but they're up. I've seen women that have small boobs, but they're like two balls just hanging down. But as I say, mine are not doing that just yet. I'm still fairly well proportioned and I wear my clothes well."

The forties seem to be a crucial bridge in our breast development that takes us into our later years—a time of adjustment and redefinition that can see us into a balanced older age or at least a less worried one. Adapting our minds to our changing bodies can be a difficult and long process in a society that so values youth. Mary Ellen, a fifty-eight-year-old journalist, explained, "As I get older they're no longer an erogenous zone because I've gone through menopause and some of the feeling isn't there anymore. There's not a great deal of use for them anymore in terms of looking good or having a lot of sex. In terms of the effects of aging, my breasts have become flatter and probably a little bit heavier as I've gained weight over the years. I'm used to it now at fifty-eight, but probably around forty-five or so, I began to see changes in my body. My waistline got a little thicker and my stomach got heavier. No matter how much walking I did, my body changed, and my breasts changed along with that. When all that was happening I was sad. My body wasn't something that I flaunted, but I was always grateful that I had a nice figure. So that began to change, but what I always tried to tell myself was, 'You're healthy, you're not going through an illness, so be grateful that you're aging in a normal way.' I do that to counteract the feelings of sadness."

Other women recognize the changes, but are more sanguine about the process. At seventy-five, Evelyn accepts the signs of aging, but she doesn't let them slow her down. An avid traveler, last year Evelyn and a friend took a two-week trip to Anarctica. "There has to be a change in my breasts as I get older. They're much smaller, they don't stand up, and they aren't firm anymore. But I think for my age, they're pretty good." Evelyn's thirty-seven-year-old daughter Shana agreed, "When I look at them now, I think they do look pretty good for your age." Evelyn continued, "I don't have the same preoccupation with my body as I did when I was younger, of course. That definitely has to change. This is the way it is and I have to cope with each age as it comes along. I wouldn't want to change my breasts or my age back."

Dr. Susan Love, author of *Dr. Susan Love's Hormone Book* in which she discusses the various options available to menopausal women, offers a powerful reminder, "One of the nice things about being a woman and going through menopause is that you have this physical wake-up call that men don't have, that says, 'You're not going to live forever. Nobody is.' It really does help you to reassess your expectations and realize that being healthy is probably the most important thing. By then you also realize that people come in all sizes and shapes and configurations and that there is no right and no normal. And we should celebrate the variations."[4] For some women, like Dr.

Love, the focus shifts from body image to health. My eighty-three-year-old grandmother admitted to being bothered by her small breasts as a younger woman, but "I don't worry about them now. They're just another part of my body. If it doesn't hurt, I don't worry about it." Lucille, seventy-six, agreed, "I don't make a big deal of my boobs. I mean they're part of my body. I don't think that much about my arms—they're just part of my body, and thank God we have arms. And thank goodness we have boobs. I was able to nurse and they make you look better in your clothes."

Older women who have lived through different eras—the flapper years, the busty fifties, the Twiggy years of the sixties, the braless look of the early seventies, and the implant boom of the eighties—have an interesting take on breast fashions. Helene, eighty-seven, reflected that it's been "a very strange journey from the end of the flapper era when flat chests were in, to our world today where women with huge breasts are a desirable physical model. I'm still affected by the early feeling that there should be some restraint in breasts. They shouldn't be allowed to proliferate indefinitely!" Lucille, seventy-six, commented on the differences between women her age and the "breast obsessed" women of younger generations. "When I was young it was different," said Lucille. "*Everything* for young people today is different. We were taught not to touch or expose ourselves. We were very sheltered. So I think there is a big difference in how one feels about her boobs."

Although Evelyn, seventy-five, has seen many changes, she feels most comfortable with the familiar attitudes of her youth. "Women have been liberated a great deal with their bodies, the way they move, the way they dress in baggy clothes. I can't get used to that because I have always emphasized my curves. And I still wear the same things I wore when I was younger, except in modern styles. When I was a girl I wore the Maidenform brassieres that made you stick out—you had to be very pointed. I had a girlfriend who knit me these very tight, short angora sweaters in beautiful bright colors, which I'd wear with straight black skirts and high heels. And I wear a lot of that even now. That's what I favor and I still emphasize the parts of the body that are sexually appealing. Maybe I just don't want to get old, I want to stay young looking. If you have it, flaunt it!"

If instead of fearing aging, we respected older women, what a different world this could be. What if a woman who had breast fed children and had older breasts was thought to be beautiful? Instead, most women are horrified when stretch marks and sagging appear, some even get surgical breast lifts. According to the American Society of Plastic and Reconstructive Surgeons, 16,097 women had breast lifts in 1996, up from 7,963 in 1992.[5] Many more women had augmentations to fill out sagging breasts, achieving the same effect as a mastopexy. Twenty-eight-year-old Judith, a mother and childbirth educator from Oklahoma, is not immune to this contempt for aging, though it makes her angry. "I have no wrinkles or lines. People comment on how young I look. But when I stand in front of the mirror, I can see my years in my breasts—they are my first sign of aging. I know that this is a normal progression of life, but it still can be a little sad. In the United States, it's boobs, boobs, and more boobs! We see boobs as a sign of youth and desire. In my Korean family, breast feeding is expected. There is honor in being a mother and having the worn breast to show for it. I like this attitude more every day."

Whether old breasts show the signs of breast feeding or simply the normal effects of living on this planet for years, we would do well to rethink our fear of aging and seek out new models of beauty in later years, and not only for our breasts. Although our breasts *do* shape our lives, the essential part of who we are is much deeper than that. What I find beautiful is strength, independence, intelligence—qualities that don't come from perky breasts and an unlined face, but from an attitude that can't help but shine through. I admire older women like Janie, Evelyn, Lucille, Helene, Penelope, and Fannie because they are so vibrant and active. And closer to my heart, as I watch my mother and grandmother grow older, I find them absolutely beautiful. I wouldn't love them more if there were no gray hairs, wrinkles, or—God forbid—sagging breasts. I hope that I can learn from them. I hope we can *all* look to older women and learn from them.

Telling Our Breast Stories

Writing this book has been a long process that has truly changed the way I think about breasts—my own and other women's. Over the past few years, I've spoken to hundreds of women and, even though there are many familiar stories, I never cease to be startled by some small detail or a twist on a common anecdote. I've often been asked what was the most surprising thing that I learned from talking to all of these women, as if there is some secret knowledge about breasts that women are hiding. Truly, there is no one great secret about breasts, but every time I did an interview or gathered together a group of women to discuss breasts, what always amazed me was just how much our breasts shape our lives, and, more than that, how eager so many women are to talk about what breasts mean to them.

In making the *Breasts* documentary and writing this book, I spoke with people I probably never would have met—women and girls of all ages, shapes, and sizes, from all over the country and from all walks of life, some of whom have very different beliefs and values from my own. And yet, I found a connection with each woman, simply because we were talking about a shared trait that is so essentially female. I laughed at some stories and was moved to tears by others. Sometimes I got angry, but most of all, hearing these women's stories forced me to examine (and reexamine) my own feelings.

My hope is that this book will do the same for you, the reader. Rather than being a passive experience, I'd love for it to trigger memories and feelings about your breasts. Perhaps you'll think of women you know and wonder what their experiences have been. Maybe you know an adolescent girl who is just developing, a new mother, or a friend or family member who is facing a health problem with her breasts. Can you imagine talking about this with your friends, sister, mother, grandmother, or your daughter? Most of us aren't used to speaking openly about these issues, so it might seem a little odd at first. To get the conversation started, you may want to mark sections of the book that you think someone else should read. (I should add that these conversations certainly aren't limited to other women—I know many women who have been inspired to talk about these issues with their husband, boyfriend, or male friends.)

When I was doing research for the book and the documentary, I used a questionnaire that asked women to "Tell Us About Your Breasts." Hundreds of women responded; and what

I found was that every woman had her own breast story. Some women filled out questionnaires on their own, others responded with a best friend, a sister, or mother, and almost all of them told me how exciting it was to consciously ask themselves these questions and think through their answers. Below is a part of the questionnaire, which you can use as a tool to explore your own breast story. Perhaps you will want to share it with a friend, family member, or colleague. I think of this as a new kind of breast self-exam. The outcome might just surprise you.

What attitudes about adult breasts did you have as a child?

When did your breasts start to develop?

Do you remember your first bra? The experience of buying it?

If you wear a bra, what kind do you prefer?

Are you satisfied with your breasts? Why or why not?

Do your breasts make you feel powerful or vulnerable? When and why?

How do you refer to your own breasts? (For example, breasts, tits, boobs.)

What comments have people made about your breasts? How has this made you feel?

What role do your breasts and nipples play in your sexual pleasure?

Have you ever had or considered having cosmetic breast surgery? Why or why not?

Have you ever breast fed? If so, what was this experience like?

Have you ever found a lump in your breast? What was the outcome?

Have breasts ever been an issue for you on the job?

How do you feel about breasts and aging?

What was your best experience involving your breasts?

What was your worst experience involving your breasts?

Describe your ideal pair of breasts.

As simple as these questions may seem, they were the starting point for the stories in this book. At first glance, you might think that you have very little to say, but simply by remembering your first bra, or the time you found a lump in your breast, or by considering what kind of physical pleasure you feel in your breasts, you are likely to uncover many stories, thoughts, and feelings.

But asking yourself these questions is just the first part of this breast self-exam. Now for the second part. Make sure that you have some privacy. Take off your shirt. Now your bra. Stand in front of a mirror. What do you see? Look at your size, your shape, your nipples, your coloring. The goal here isn't to search for problems—it's to step back for a moment and see your breasts in a new way. What stories do your breasts tell? (I say "breasts," but the same goes if you've had a lumpectomy or mastectomy.)

So what do we do with this information? This knowledge can be powerful if we use it to form a deeper understanding of what our breasts mean to us. And with this understanding, come to accept and love them. After hearing all of these women's stories, my own worries about the size of my breasts disappeared—my hope is that you will have your own breast breakthrough. I know that the women who shared their stories told me that speaking about these issues allowed them to feel freer about their bodies. One woman who had a mastectomy said that doing the interview allowed her to talk to her friends for the first time about losing her breast to cancer. I'd love for this kind of exploration and honesty to become commonplace instead of remarkable.

I believe that we owe ourselves the chance to know our bodies better. Most of us recognize the importance of understanding our psychology, soul, and mind, so why are our breasts any less important? Our breasts have something to tell us . . . all we have to do is listen.

Endnotes

Childhood

1. M. G. Lord, *Forever Barbie: The Unauthorized Biography of a Real Doll* (New York: William Morrow and Company, Inc., 1994), 9.

Puberty

1. Judy Blume, *Are You There God? It's Me Margaret* (New York: Bantam Doubleday Dell, 1970), 37.
2. *Seventeen* magazine, October 1964, 134.
3. Simone de Beauvoir, *The Second Sex*, trans. and ed. H. M. Parshley (New York: Knopf, 1971), 287.
4. Women's Health Special Section, *New York Times*, 21 June 1998, 28.
5. Ibid.

Identity

1. Nora Ephron, "A Few Words About Breasts" in *Crazy Salad: Some Things About Women* (New York: Knopf, 1975), 11-12. Originally published in *Esquire* magazine, May 1972.
2. Dr. Susan Love, telephone interview with author, New York, NY, 20 May 1998.
3. This information was retrieved from the American Society of Plastic and Reconstructive Surgeons website: www. plasticsurgery.org, July 1998.
4. Ibid.
5. Ibid.

Sexuality

1. Dr. Theodore Van de Velde, *Ideal Marriage: Its Physiology*

and Technique (New York: Random House, 1926), 164.

2. Ibid., 45.

3. June M. Reinisch, Ph.D., with Ruth Beasley, MLS, *The Kinsey Institute New Report on Sex: What You Must Know to Be Sexually Literate* (New York: St. Martin's Press, 1990), 67.

Motherhood

1. H. Newcome, *The compleat mother, or An earnest persuasive to all mothers to nurse their own children* (London, 1695), quoted in Valerie A. Fildes, *Breasts, Bottles and Babies: A History of Infant Feeding* (Edinburgh: Edinburgh University Press, 1986), 106.

2. Anna Freud, *The Harvard Lectures*, ed. Joseph Sandler (London: The Institute of Psycho-Analysis, Karnac Books, 1992).

Health

1. Susan Love, M.D., with Karen Lindsey, *Dr. Susan Love's Breast Book*, 2d ed. (New York: Addison Wesley, 1995), xxviii.

2. Love, interview.

3. Miriam Stoppard, M.D., *The Breast Book: The Essential Guide to Breast Care and Breast Health for Women of All Ages* (New York: DK Publishing, 1996), 116-118.

4. Love, *Breast Book,* 109.

5. Love, interview.

6. Ibid.

7. Front Page, *New York Times,* 9 July 1998.

8. Love, interview.

9. This information was retrieved from the American Cancer Society website: www.cancer.org, July 1998.

10. Ibid.

11. Love, interview.

12. American Cancer Society website, *Cancer Risk Report, 1995:* "The Society recommends that screening mammograms should begin by age 40. Women 40 to 49 should have a mammogram every 1-2 years; women 50 and older should have a mammogram every year."

—National Cancer Institute website, www.nci.nih.gov, August 1998, *Cancer Facts: Screening Mammograms:* "The National Cancer Institute recommends that women in their forties or older get screening mammograms on a regular basis, every 1 to 2 years."

—Love, *Breast Book,* 259: "What I recommend is doing a 'baseline' mammogram in your early 40s to find out what your breast tissue looks like. . . . Once you're in your 50s (or whenever your breast density makes it feasible), you should have regular mammograms, every year or two."

13. Love, *Breast Book,* 255.

14. Ibid., 258.

15. This information was retrieved from the National Alliance of Breast Cancer Organizations website: www.nabco.org, July 1998.

16. Love, interview.

17. American Cancer Society, website.

18. Ibid.

19. Love, interview.

Aging

1. Autumn Stephens, ed., *Wild Words from Wild Women: An Unbridled Collection of Candid Observations and Extremely Opinionated Bon Mots* (Berkeley: Conari Press, 1993), 247.

2. Betty Friedan, *The Fountain of Age* (New York: Simon & Schuster, 1993).

3. Stoppard, *The Breast Book,* 43.

4. Love, interview.

5. American Society of Plastic and Reconstructive Surgeons, website.

About the Author

Meema Spadola is an award-winning producer, director, and writer of film, television, and radio, living in New York City. *Breasts* is her first book. Her documentary *Breasts* began as an independent production and was the highest rated program ever aired on the Cinemax series "Reel Life." HBO has since commissioned Spadola and *Breasts* co-producer Thom Powers to make a documentary about men and their penises, which will air in 1999.

In addition, she has produced and written radio documentaries for the Peabody Award-winning public radio show "This American Life." Spadola's short documentary "My Mother's Secret" about children of lesbian mothers was shown at film festivals around the world. In the coming year, she will be producing and directing an hour-long documentary about children of gay parents for public television. She also produced live segments for "Breakfast Time" on Fox Television's fX cable network, and has worked as an associate producer, researcher, and assistant editor on a variety of films.

Spadola grew up in Searsmont, Maine, studied in Paris, and graduated from Sarah Lawrence College in 1992.

Tell Us About Your Breasts

Do you want to share your breast story? Send it to the address on the following page and be sure to include your name, address, and phone number. We will contact you if we decide it is appropriate for any new editions of the book.

• • • • •

Wildcat Canyon Press publishes books that embrace such subjects as friendship, spirituality, women's issues, and home and family, all with a focus on self-help and personal growth. Great care is taken to create books that inspire reflection and improve the quality of our lives. Our books invite sharing and are frequently given as gifts.

For a catalog of our publications, please write:

WILDCAT CANYON PRESS
2716 Ninth Street
Berkeley, California 94710
Phone: (510) 848-3600
Fax: (510) 848-1326
Circulus@aol.com

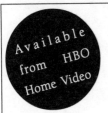
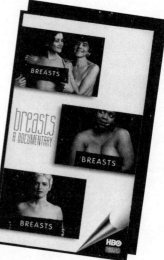